Heart Attacks,

Heart Failure,

and

Diabetes

Prevention and Treatment

Mark Starr MD(H)

Mark Starr Trust

Starr, Mark
Heart Attacks, Heart Failure, and Diabetes: Prevention and Treatment

ISBN:	978-0-9913688-0-8
LCCN:	2013958160
Published by:	Mark Starr Trust
	Scottsdale, AZ
	www.21centurymed.com

Dedication

I dedicate this book to Broda O. Barnes M.D., Ph.D. and to his research foundation (brodabarnes.org). Telephone 203 261-2101 USA.

Acknowledgements

For helping edit the final drafts of this book, many thanks to my dear sister Dr. Sydney Starr, Ivan Danhof, M.D., Ph.D., and my editor Marcus Plourde, Ph.D. Many thanks to my brother Steven Starr for his research and contributions.

TABLE OF CONTENTS

LIST OF TABLES AND FIGURES

TABLES

FIGURES

When medical treatments do not make sense

the answer is always dollars and cents.

— Mark Starr

Introduction

Health care is hands down the most profitable business on our planet. Currently, health care costs are estimated to be about 18% of America's gross domestic gross domestic production (dwarfing military expenditures of 4.4%). According to a study published in the journal entitled *Circulation*, the cost to treat heart disease in the United States will triple by the year 2030. Currently, one in three Americans have some form of heart disease, including high blood pressure, coronary heart disease, heart failure, stroke, and other conditions. The estimated costs for medical treatments related to heart disease in 2008 were $273 billion. The American Heart Association projects those costs will rise to $818 billion by the year 2030.[1]

The cause of heart attacks and how to prevent them from occurring was conclusively established when Broda Barnes M.D., Ph.D. endocrinologist published his book entitled *Solved: The Riddle of Heart Attacks* in 1976. His research proved that hypothyroidism was the underlying cause of heart attacks and proper treatment for hypothyroidism prevented heart attacks. Dr. Barnes' book is now out of print but copies remain available from his research foundation.

Dr. Barnes received a Masters Degree in Biochemistry at Case Western Reserve University in 1930, followed by a Ph.D. in Physiology from the University of Chicago in 1931. He specialized in physiology of the thyroid gland for his doctorate. He continued thyroid research for the next five years while teaching endocrinology before obtaining his medical degree from Rush Medical College in 1937. The rest of his life was devoted to treating patients and doing clinical and scientific research with regard to the thyroid related illnesses. Dr. Barnes died in 1988 at the age of 82.

Heart Attacks,

Heart Failure,

and

Diabetes

Prevention and Treatment

Chapter 1
Heart Attacks:
Prevention and Treatment

The thyroid gland is shaped like a butterfly and is situated just below the Adam's apple. Hormones produced from this endocrine gland are responsible for our metabolism. Metabolism is the sum of all physical and chemical processes by which living substances are produced and maintained. Metabolism is the transformation by which energy is made available for the uses of the organism. In simple terms, thyroid hormones control the efficiency and speed at which all of our cells work.

> Of all your hormones, the thyroid is the most important!

Without the crucial influence of thyroid hormones, proper maturation and function of the other hormone glands is not possible. Thyroid hormones both stimulate the cellular energy production necessary for life, as well as maintain our body's relatively constant temperature. The thyroid orchestrates the development of our brain and sexual maturation. Thyroid hormones stimulate synthesis of the protein building blocks that are necessary to replenish the constant turnover of trillions of cells. They are necessary for growth and to keep us healthy. Harmful cellular waste products accumulate without proper thyroid function. The immune system is dynamic, energy intensive, and dependent upon normal thyroid function. **Susceptibility to infection is one of the hallmarks of hypothyroidism (low thyroid function).** No matter what you eat or how much you exercise, your health will suffer without proper thyroid function.

Appendix A provides a list of the known physiological functions of thyroid hormones.

History of Hypothyroidism

In 1875, Sir William Gull presented the first case reports of hypothyroidism in adults to The Clinical Society of London.

The association between damaged arteries and hypothyroidism was first noted in an 1877 autopsy report by Dr. William Ord. A middle-aged woman had died and Dr. Ord performed an autopsy to investigate why the woman had died. Upon cutting into her skin, he saw tissues that were thickened and boggy. Her tissues appeared to be waterlogged but no water seeped from his incisions. Dr. Ord realized this disease was unique and previously unrecognized. Dr. Ord summoned a leading chemist to help identify the substance that was causing the woman's tissues to be boggy. What they found was an abnormally large accumulation of mucin.

Mucin is a normal constituent of our tissues. It is a jellylike material that spontaneously accumulates in hypothyroidism. Mucin grabs onto water and causes firm swelling. Fifty times the normal amount of mucin was found in the woman's skin. Her other tissues also contained excess mucin. Dr. Ord named the previously unknown illness "myxedema."

Myx is the Greek word for mucin and edema means swelling. Myxedema was adopted as the medical term for hypothyroidism (myxedema and hypothyroidism are one and the same entity).

The edema or swelling associated with hypothyroidism usually begins around the face, particularly above or below the eyes and along the jawline. However, the skin on the side of the upper arms may be thickened early in the course of the disease. The swelling associated with hypothyroidism is firm and will eventually spread throughout the body's connective tissues.

One of the many functions of connective tissue is to help hold our body's organs and structures together. Connective tissue lines our blood vessels, nervous system, muscles, mucous membranes such as the sinuses, the gut, as well as each and every cell in our glands and organs. Abnormal accumulation of mucin in these tissues causes swelling and significantly impairs normal functioning. This type of swelling is unique to hypothyroidism. Medical textbooks about hypothyroidism state that myxedema is thyroprival (pertaining to or characterized by hypothyroidism) and pathognomonic (specifically distinctive and diagnostic).

Translation: If the thickened skin or myxedema is present, you have hypothyroidism.

The first comprehensive report on the subject of myxedema (hypothyroidism) was published in 1888 by The Clinical Society of London. The following quote was taken from this research paper. **"The general uniformity of the more prominent symptoms is, indeed, remarkable, allowing ready recognition of the malady in any freshly encountered case by an observer who has seen one well pronounced case."**

Doctors no longer recognize "the general uniformity of the most prominent symptoms."

The following illustrations are from the Report of the Committee of the Clinical Society of London to investigate the subject of myxedema.

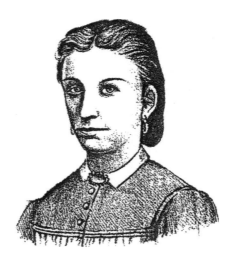

Before myxedema
age 21

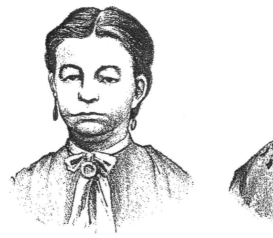

Mild myxedema
age 28

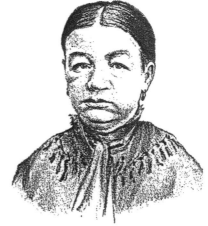

Marked myxedema
age 32

Source: The Clinical Society of London. Report of the Committee of
the Clinical Society of London to investigate the subject of
myxoedema. *Trans Clinical Soc London*. 1888. Supp. Vol. 21.

The first illustration is of the woman at age 21, prior to the onset of hypothyroidism. A second illustration at age 28, shows puffiness accumulating along her jawline as well as puffiness in her eyelids. Her lips are turning down, which is another common finding in hypothyroidism. The third illustration, four years later at age 32, shows the common features of a well-pronounced case. Such a case should be recognized immediately according to the 1888 report.

A flurry of research followed the 1888 report. Doctors began removing thyroid glands from animals to study the consequences. Greatly accelerated atherosclerosis (hardening of the arteries) occurred after removal of the thyroid gland in all of the different animals studied. Administering thyroid glands halted the progression of atherosclerosis. The first cure of a person who suffered from hypothyroidism was in 1891.

By 1915, medical textbooks contained pictures of hypothyroid patients before treatment and after treatment. I have included photographs from an article authored by the first generation Hertoghe endocrinologist (although the term endocrinologist had not yet been coined). The fourth generation Hertoghe endocrinologist continues to practice in Belgium.

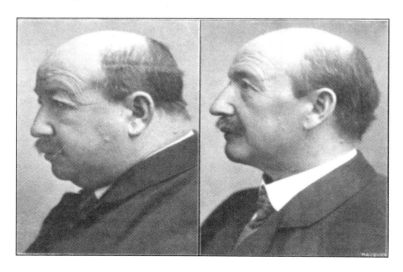

Before Treatment   After Treatment

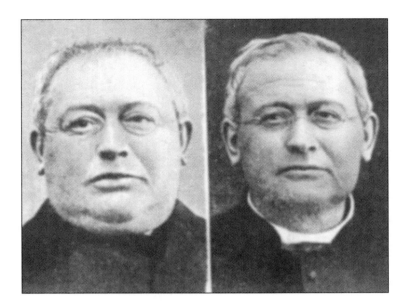

Before treatment   After treatment

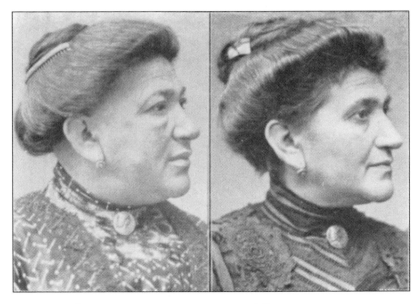

Before treatment   After treatment

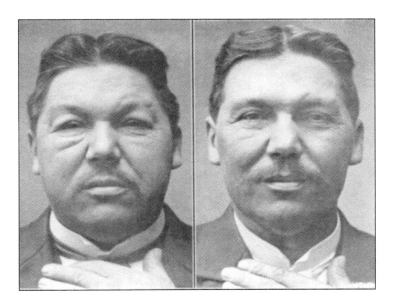

Before treatment   After treatment

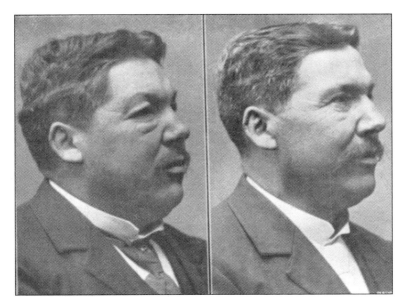

Before treatment   After treatment

Source: Hertoghe E. *The Practitioner*. Vol XCIV No 1. Jan 1915. Pages 26-69.

Proper treatment usually resolves the myxedema. However, only slightly more than half of people who have hypothyroidism will ever develop myxedema or puffiness. Many do so as they age.

More than one hundred different symptoms may be associated with hypothyroidism. Opposite symptoms such as very short stature or very tall stature, hyperactivity or profound fatigue, being underweight or obese, are just a few examples. The insidious nature of onset, as well as myriad possible symptoms, has made hypothyroidism difficult for doctors to diagnose.

Dr. Barnes believed recurrent infections, which are often associated with hypothyroidism, to be largely responsible for the accelerated atherosclerosis. Infections cause inflammation and can damage the lining of our arteries. He cited autopsy studies from 1969 that showed evidence of atherosclerosis in all of the children who had died by age three, whether they were from third world countries or modernized nations.[2]

At the University of Chicago in the 1930s, Dr. Barnes removed the thyroid glands of baby rabbits to demonstrate to his students the physiological changes of hypothyroidism. The rabbits' life span was halved and most of the physical changes associated with hypothyroidism, including recurrent infections and markedly accelerated arterial damage were demonstrable. Dr. Barnes published research studies showing the restoration of normal immune function after giving proper thyroid hormones.[3]

A large percentage of my patients suffered recurrent infections before they were treated for their hypothyroidism. Following proper treatment, their immune system was restored and they no longer suffered from infections.[3] **Susceptibility to infections and accelerated atherosclerosis are hallmarks of hypothyroidism.**

Some of the most common symptoms of hypothyroidism include fatigue and weakness, cold intolerance, joint and muscle pain, headaches and migraines, depression, obesity, muscle cramps, dry skin that is often puffy, constipation, chronic dental problems, and numerous other symptoms such as acne, premature aging with parchment like wrinkles, and a whole host of mental problems.

Menstrual problems such as heavy bleeding, irregular cycles, severe cramping, as well as infertility are hallmarks of hypothyroidism.

When my practice was located in Atlanta (GA), my office manager advised me to have younger female patients sign a release that would exempt me from any liability with regard to pregnancies. Why? Proper treatment for hypothyroidism markedly improves fertility. Many patients would become pregnant shortly after beginning thyroid hormones. Numerous older female patients that I have treated had problems with infertility when they were young. Gynecologists and primary care doctors used to prescribe desiccated thyroid for infertile women (for the first half of the 20th century). Most of these women had several healthy babies shortly thereafter.

Children are almost always born with hypothyroidism, if their mother suffered from hypothyroidism throughout her pregnancy. Numerous complications may occur including prematurity, hemorrhaging, preeclampsia, excessive weight gain, gestational diabetes, and other problems during delivery such as inability to dilate. Postpartum problems such as depression, fatigue, and inability to breast feed may also result if the mother suffers hypothyroidism.

Long-term consequences include heart attack and congestive heart failure, high blood pressure, sleep apnea, carpal tunnel syndrome, high cholesterol, menstrual difficulties, increased risk of cancer, diabetes, and autoimmune disorders such as Hashimoto's thyroiditis (when the body attacks its own thyroid gland) and goiters.

Hypothyroidism's Connection to Heart Attacks

Dr. Barnes believed hypothyroidism was the underlying cause of the tremendous increase in heart attacks during the 20th century. The etiology or cause of heart attacks was not described until 1912. Dr. Barnes noted from his medical school training in the early 1930s that heart attacks were a minor problem at that time. Heart attacks were extremely rare among his large group of patients being treated for hypothyroidism. Yet, they were increasing dramatically in the general population during the late 1940s.

Dr. Barnes made a serendipitous discovery through the American Medical Society of Vienna. Empress Maria Theresa, renowned 18th century monarch of Austria, passed a law that mandated autopsies be performed on all hospital deaths occurring in Graz, Austria. The state of health was terrible in Graz at that time. About 75% of the total deaths were autopsied each year, which was more than enough to establish any changes in the patterns of deaths over time.

In the early 18th century, doctors began to correlate clinical symptoms and physical examination with postmortem findings at the autopsy. Autopsy developed into an essential routine at the great medical centers. Only then did medicine slowly emerge from the archaic belief in humoralism, put forth over fourteen centuries earlier. Humoralism was the ancient theory that health and illness resulted from a balance or imbalance of bodily liquids (humors). One of the most common treatments associated with this practice was bloodletting. In 1827, 33 million leeches were imported into France.

Dr. Barnes hoped to prove the cause of heart attacks by studying these autopsies. Beginning in 1958, and stretching into the 1970s, Dr. Barnes spent every summer studying the autopsies. From the first 10,000 autopsies, Dr. Barnes found only one person who was not suffering some degree of atherosclerosis. This included the very young who succumbed to infections and cancer. The autopsies revealed only one heart attack per 125 deaths occurred in 1930. By 1970 heart attacks had increased to one death in 14. This came about with little change in the Austrian's diet, which was similar to the American diet during that time.

Dr. Barnes published the autopsy results in a paper entitled "The Role of Natural Consequences in the Changing Death Patterns." The comparisons from the autopsy results are listed in Table 1. Note the numbers of deaths are per 1000 autopsies.

Table 1

Phenomenal Rise In the Incidence of a Few Diseases According to Autopsies at Graz, Austria, Between 1930 and 1970 (number per 1,000 autopsies)

Category	1930	1970	% Change
Heart attacks	6.8	69.0	+915
Emphysema	8.6	40.6	+372
Prostatic cancer	1.8	8.3	+361
Cancer in children	1.2	5.4	+349
Bronchial (lung) cancer	11.0	44.0	+300

Table 2

Fluctuations In Various Categories of Deaths at Graz, Austria, 1930 and 1970 (number per 1,000 autopsies)

Category	1930	1970	% Change
Deaths from infections	426	185	−56
Deaths from malignancies	189	240	+27
Deaths from degenerative diseases	238	343	+44
Deaths from accidents	37	47	+27

Source: Barnes B, Ratzenhofer M, Gisi R. The role of natural consequences in changing death patterns. *J Am Geriatr Soc.* 1974; 22(4):176-179. Reprinted with permission.

Table 2 shows that over 42% (426 per 1,000) of the deaths in 1930 resulted from infectious diseases. By 1970, deaths from infections had fallen to 18% (185 per 1,000) of the total. Those patients, who were susceptible to infections, were now surviving long enough to develop heart attacks, emphysema, malignancies, and other degenerative diseases.

The autopsies revealed that in 1930, only 47% of the total deaths were from patients over 50 years old. By 1970, total deaths for those over the age of 50 were 67%.

Historically, patients who contracted tuberculosis (TB) were 20 times more likely to develop lung cancer than the general population. Eradicating tuberculosis allowed those who were susceptible to infectious diseases time enough to develop lung cancer. This explains why so many people who have never smoked cigarettes may have developed lung cancer.

> The rate of the increase in heart attacks paralleled the drop of deaths caused by infections.

Prior to the introduction of antituberculin drugs in 1944, the average age of death for tuberculosis victims was 38 years. The average age for first heart attacks has remained in the 60s since becoming public enemy number one.

In 1870, deaths from tuberculosis in America had been 270 per 100,000. By 1900, sanatoria care (hospitals specifically caring for tuberculosis) resulted in the number of deaths from TB to be halved. For the first time, people who were susceptible to infections were able to survive. For thousands of years, smallpox had eliminated many of those who were susceptible to infections. After Dr. Jenner pioneered the vaccinations that would eliminate smallpox, tuberculosis became the number one killer.

Antibiotics and antituberculin drugs were introduced to the general population in 1944. A year by year study of the autopsies revealed very little change in death patterns until the introduction of antibiotics and antituberculin drugs to the general populace, which began after the invasion of Normandy in 1944 during World War II. Therefore, most of these dramatic changes in death patterns occurred in only 25 years (1945-1970).

The comparisons of death categories from autopsy results are listed in Table 2. The frequency of heart attacks had risen over 900% (Table 1), thanks to the elimination of tuberculosis and infections through the usage of antibiotics and antituberculin drugs.

The rate of heart attacks dropped precipitously in Europe during World War II, and Graz was no exception. Most scientists and doctors attributed the decline to the wartime diet, which was low in animal fats and dairy products (i.e., low cholesterol). I will explain how the autopsies proved their theory wrong.

The incidence of heart attacks in 1939, at the start of the war, was 12 per 1000 autopsies. By 1945, there were only three deaths from heart attacks per 1000. However, atherosclerosis in the aorta (our largest artery originating from the heart) and the blood vessels supplying the heart (coronary arteries) had doubled in severity among autopsied patients under the age of 50. The number of patients affected with atherosclerosis under the age of 50 had also doubled. In other words, atherosclerosis had quadrupled in only six years. The elimination of animal fats and dairy products appeared to greatly accelerate atherosclerosis.

If atherosclerosis was accelerated, then why the drop in heart attacks? In 1939, there were 27 deaths from tuberculosis per 1000 men between 30 and 60 years of age. In 1944 there were 55 deaths from tuberculosis per 1000. Deaths from other infections also rose. The deaths from tuberculosis and other infections accounted for the drop from 12 to three deaths from heart attacks per 1000 autopsies. Germany had a precipitous rise in tuberculosis during the war and a marked decline in heart attacks. Great Britain had a slight increase in tuberculosis and a slight decrease in heart attacks during the war. TB and infections did not increase in America, thus heart attacks did not decline. Penicillin and antituberculin drugs were introduced in 1944, extending the life of patients. Heart attacks spiraled upward.

Can you guess what the autopsies from 1944 and 1945 revealed about the coronary arteries from those who died from tuberculosis? Severe atherosclerosis is correct. The Graz autopsies revealed advanced atherosclerosis in all of the patients who died from tuberculosis. Had they not died from TB, a heart attack likely would have ensued.

What do you think the 1947 autopsies revealed about those now dying from heart attacks? Their lungs were full of tuberculosis.

> The low cholesterol wartime diet decreased immunity and markedly accelerated atherosclerosis.

By 1950, Dr. Barnes recognized that his patients had not suffered any heart attacks while their incidence was exploding in the rest of America. He began a long-term study to determine if proper treatment for hypothyroidism would prevent heart attacks.

The National Heart Institute had begun a large study in 1948. It was called the Framingham Study, but was officially named "The Heart Disease Epidemiology Study." Its objective was to determine why heart attacks were rapidly reaching epidemic proportions.

Over 5,000 adult residents of Framingham, Massachusetts volunteered to participate in the long term medical study. The group underwent thorough physical exams. All were free of heart disease initially. Participants were examined at two-year intervals. People who later suffered heart attacks helped to determine the so-called risk factors. Risk factors included high blood pressure, elevated cholesterol, increasing age, and having a family history of heart attacks. Men were found to be at higher risk of heart attacks than women.

Dr. Barnes intended for his study to parallel the Framingham Study. Data from the ongoing Framingham Study was published every few years. In 1976, Dr. Barnes published the results of his work in a book entitled *Hypothyroidism, the Unsuspected Illness*.[4] Table 3 compared his findings to those from the Framingham Study.

Table 3

Comparison of the Framingham Study
Prediction of Heart Attacks versus Dr. Barnes' Actual Cases

Sex	Classification	# of Patients Treated	Patient Years	Framingham Coronary Prediction	Barnes' Actual Cases
F	Age 30-59	490	2,705	7.6	0
F	High risk*	172	1,086	7.3	0
F	Age over 60	182	955	7.8	0
M	Age 30-59	382	2,192	12.8	1
M	High risk*	186	1,070	18.5	2
M	Age over 60	157	816	18.0	1
	Totals	1,569	8,824	72.0	4

*High risk = high cholesterol, high blood pressure, or both.

Source: Barnes B. *Hypothyroidism, the Unsuspected Illness*, Harper and Row, 1976; page 180. Reprinted with permission.

Over 90% of predicted heart attacks from the Framingham Study were prevented.

Dr. Barnes research included 1,569 patients who received treatment for their hypothyroidism. A minimum of two years of thyroid therapy was required to be included in the study. A number of these patients had been on thyroid medication for the entire study. An individual patient's symptoms, the patient's response to the thyroid hormones, and basal temperatures determined their dosage of desiccated thyroid hormones.

The chart shows the comparison between his patients and those from the Framingham Study. The Framingham Study would have predicted that 72 of Dr. Barnes' patients should have suffered heart attacks. **Only four heart attacks occurred. Thirty patients who quit the study and discontinued thyroid hormones suffered a fatal heart attack within six years of stopping their thyroid.** Many of these patients had moved. Their new doctors may have declined to continue thyroid treatment. Blood tests often showed that these patients did not need thyroid hormones.

Others stopped taking their medication after their symptoms, such as acne resolved. Dr. Barnes purposely did not attempt to control cholesterol, smoking, exercise, or other variables among his study group. He wanted the only variable between his patients and those from the Framingham Study, to be the usage of thyroid hormones.

Changing Death Patterns Not Related to Diet

Drs. Barnes' and Ratzenhofer's paper, "The Role of Natural Consequences in the Changing Death Patterns," included a listing from the World Health Organization (WHO) on the distribution of the sexes in deaths from tuberculosis for the years 1947 to 1949 in several countries.

Table 4   **WHO - TB Deaths from 1947 - 1949**

		per 100,000
Country	Males	Females
Japan	169	129
Italy	59	38
England	53	33
Canada	34	28
U.S. (whites)	30	14

Source: Barnes B, Ratzenhofer M, Gisi R. The role of natural consequences in changing death patterns. *J Am Geriatr Soc.* 1974; 22(4):176-179. Reprinted with permission.

This shows us that the Asian hypothyroid population was dying from tuberculosis and other infections just like those from Graz in 1930. Thanks to TB, they did not live long enough to develop lethal coronary artery disease. Therefore, the lower incidence of heart attacks almost certainly did not result from their diet.

Dr. Barnes made special note in his research and lecture tapes regarding the lack of heart attacks in underprivileged third world countries. Without exception, deaths from infectious diseases accounted for the scarcity of heart attacks. The bibliographies from his books list many such studies that included autopsy findings.

Drs. Barnes and Ratzenhofer concluded their research paper by stating:

"It is fitting that the tuberculosis sanatoriums of the past are being converted into general hospitals for the management of heart attacks. The identical patients are being cared for, but they are arriving 25 years later with a new ailment."[5]

For the first half of the 20th century, desiccated thyroid was the mainstream treatment for hypothyroidism. Desiccated thyroid is a dried glandular thyroid from pigs' thyroid glands. It was called Armour thyroid, which was produced by the Armour meat packing company. Desiccated Armour thyroid was first produced in the early 1900s. Gunpowder was measured in grains, and so was desiccated thyroid. One grain of desiccated thyroid weighs approximately 65 mg. The dosages used in Dr. Barnes study group ranged from 2 to 5 grains daily. All four patients who had suffered heart attacks were on the minimum dosage of 2 grains. Dr. Barnes thought that had he paid more attention to those four patients and raised their dosages slightly, his study group may not have had any heart attacks.

Lectures by Dr. Barnes regarding his research are available through his foundation. He was in his 70s in the 1970s when the lectures were recorded. After lecturing, he fielded questions from the doctors in his audience. One doctor asked him if his patients ever died. Dr. Barnes stated that strokes were the most common cause of death in his treatment group. However, most of his patients were living into their 80s and 90s with all of their faculties intact. There were no cases of dementia or Alzheimer's disease. There were no cases of congestive heart failure. In addition, over 100 patients entered the study with a prior diagnosis of high blood pressure. About 80% of the patients with high blood pressure were completely relieved of their blood pressure problem just by taking thyroid hormones. In addition, there were no cases of chronic kidney failure. The occurrence of new cases of diabetes was quite rare. Diabetes had already begun to increase rapidly in the rest of America.

Barnes' Monumental Research Is Ignored

The *Townsend Letter* is one of the leading integrative medicine journals that offers alternatives to standard treatments such as prescription drugs. A rapidly growing number of doctors are prescribing nutrition and other alternative treatments. The *Townsend Letter* published a recent journal devoted to the treatment of heart disease and heart attacks. There was no mention of Dr. Barnes' research. What follows is my letter to the editor.

Dear Townsend Editors,

I was very disappointed after reading the May 2013 *Townsend Letter*. Cardiovascular health and heart attacks were the topics of discussion. There was no mention of the mountain of research performed by Broda Barnes M.D., Ph.D. regarding heart attacks. His research Foundation has been carrying his torch since his death in 1988 (brodabarnes.org).

Dr. Barnes was an endocrinologist who knew that accelerated hardening of the arteries and low immune function were hallmarks of hypothyroidism. His first book, *Hypothyroidism; the Unsuspected Illness*, was published in 1976. Included in the book was a 22 year study on heart attacks within his patient population. His study paralleled the Framingham Study.

In 1972, Dr. Barnes published his results after 22 years of research involving 1,569 patients. A minimum of two years thyroid therapy was required to be included in the study. A number of patients were followed throughout the study. At the time of the publication, there had been 8,824 patient treatment years.

The Framingham Study would have predicted that 72 of Dr. Barnes' patients should have suffered heart attacks. Only four occurred. In addition, at least 30 patients who quit the study and discontinued thyroid hormones suffered fatal heart attacks within six years of stopping their thyroid.

All four patients who suffered heart attacks were taking 2 grains of thyroid. Dr. Barnes theorized that had he increased these patient's dosages, there may not have been any heart attacks in his study group.

By giving his patients desiccated thyroid (dosages ranging from 2 grains to 5 grains of desiccated thyroid) he prevented over 90% of predicted heart attacks. He did not attempt to control cholesterol, smoking, exercise, or any other variables among his study group.

His landmark book entitled: *Solved: The Riddle of Heart Attacks* was also published in 1976. Having read all four of his books and having listened to his lectures, my goal has been to increase my adult patient's thyroid replacement dosages to more than 2 grains of thyroid or the equivalent dosage of compounded T4 and T3 (T4-76 mcg and T3-18 mcg).

I have treated over 1,500 hypothyroid patients since learning about Dr. Barnes research. The vast majority of my patients are chronically ill and many are elderly. **None of my patients on more than 2 grains of thyroid or the equivalent has ever had a heart attack.**

Dr. Barnes also determined that anyone who has already had a heart attack will not tolerate more than 2 grains of desiccated thyroid or its equivalent T4-76 mcg / T3-18 mcg). I have found that to be invariably correct.

It is a sad commentary that Dr. Barnes' research languishes and is not taught in any medical school or accredited training program. I find it astonishing and disappointing that the *Townsend Letter* also chooses to ignore his monumental research.

Mark Starr M.D.(H)

Townsend Letter References

Barnes B., Galton L. *Hypothyroidism: The Unsuspected Illness.* New York: Harper and Row Publishers; 1976.

Barnes B.O. *Heart Attack Rareness in Thyroid–Treated Patients.* Springfield, IL: Charles C. Thomas. 1972.

Barnes B.O. *Solved: The Riddle of Heart Attacks.* Trumbull, CT: The Broda O. Barnes M.D. Research Foundation. 1976.

Barnes B.O. *Thyroid Therapy I, II, III* (Audio Tapes). Copies are available through The Broda O. Barnes M.D. Research Foundation (www.brodabarnes.org).

Starr M. *Hypothyroidism Type 2: The Epidemic.* New Voice Publications, Irvine, CA. 2005, revised 2013.

Published in *Townsend Letter* August / September 2013.

My Clinical Experience

I was very fortunate to learn about Dr. Barnes' research very early in my medical career. It has been my goal to gradually raise adults' dosages of desiccated thyroid above the 2 grains threshold.

None of the adult patients whom I have treated with more than 2 grains of desiccated thyroid (or the equivalent dosages of compounded T4 and T3 (which are the synthetic forms of thyroid hormones) have ever had a heart attack. It appears that Dr. Barnes was correct in presuming that using more than 2 grains of desiccated thyroid eliminates heart attacks and stops the progression of atherosclerosis.

Four patients of mine did suffer heart attacks shortly after beginning desiccated thyroid hormones. Thyroid hormones are one of the most powerful natural medications that a doctor can prescribe. When given relatively small dosages, patients' hearts begin to beat more forcefully, which means the heart requires additional blood flow through its arteries. If the heart's arteries (coronary arteries) have arterial sclerosis or hardening of the arteries, and the heart is unable to obtain the increased blood flow it requires, a heart attack may ensue. Please read Chapter 4 carefully in order to avoid heart attacks when beginning treatment with thyroid hormones.

Addendum

Several days prior to the publication of this book, a 56 year-old male patient of mine had a heart attack. He already had a history of coronary artery disease (arterial sclerosis), sleep apnea, fatigue, insomnia, and severe dental problems. Two coronary arterial stents had been placed at age 40. Two more stents were placed at age 50. After his initial visit two years ago, I slowly increased his thyroid dosages over a lengthy period of time. He also required a small dosage of prednisone to correct mild adrenal deficiency. Most of his symptoms resolved, but he still suffered from sleep apnea.

He was taking T4-133 mcg and T3-31.5 mcg per day (the equivalent of 3.5 grains) plus 5 mg of prednisone when he had his heart attack.

He was admitted to the hospital the previous day after he complained of shortness of breath and tightness in his chest. The heart attack occurred while in the hospital at 5 AM. He was scheduled to have a stress test the next morning.

After his heart attack, the cardiac catheterization showed minimal plaque. However, he had complete blockage of the right main coronary artery. Two stents had previously been placed in the right main coronary artery. The stents were adjacent to the blocked artery that caused his heart attack. Three more stents were added in the affected artery and he was discharged two days later.

I saw this patient four days after his heart attack. He was doing very well and his only symptom was mild to moderate fatigue. I reduced his dosage of thyroid to 1.5 grains per day, and instructed him to begin 2 grains per day one month later. The next day, he was cleared for light duty work.

Chapter 2
Congestive Heart Failure:
Prevention and Treatment

The American Heart Association estimates current costs of heart failure are $31 billion a year. They project the costs could reach $160 billion by the year 2030.[6]

Over five million Americans currently suffer from congestive heart failure or CHF. More than 500,000 new cases are diagnosed each year. Fifty percent of patients die within five years of their initial diagnosis.[7]

People who suffer CHF usually have a gradual decline in their health as the heart begins to fail. Right-sided heart failure results in swelling in the feet and ankles, legs, and abdominal organs. Left-sided heart failure usually involves swelling and congestion in the lungs accompanied with difficulty breathing.

After completing my residency training at the Howard A. Rusk Rehabilitation Center in Columbia (MO), I spent two years of additional study in New York City. At that time I had the incredible opportunity to work with Dr. Lawrence S. Sonkin, M.D., Ph.D. endocrinologist. Dr. Sonkin taught me his method for treating hypothyroidism. After opening my pain clinic in Columbia, I began to suffer ridicule from my colleagues because Dr. Sonkin taught me to treat patients' symptoms instead of the TSH thyroid blood test, which he thought to be erroneous.

As a result, I decided to comb the medical literature in an attempt to understand how treatment for hypothyroidism had gone so wrong. I spent six years searching through medical textbooks and journals that were old and relegated to library storage.

Dr. Broda Barnes authored four books, all of which were very well referenced.[8] "Well referenced" means that all of his literature and medical studies were properly noted. This allows researchers to investigate how he reached his conclusions. His references were wonderful starting points for me to find excellent information concerning clinical treatments for hypothyroidism.

In 1918, Dr. Hermann Zondek was the first to report that proper treatment for hypothyroidism resolved congestive heart failure. He published the following X-rays showing a heart shrinking to normal size within weeks of beginning treatment with desiccated thyroid. The patient's symptoms associated with heart failure and hypothyroidism resolved. The black shadow in the middle of the X-ray is the heart. The white area shows the lungs and ribs. The upper left X-ray shows an enlarged heart. The bottom X-ray shows that the size of the heart has normalized.

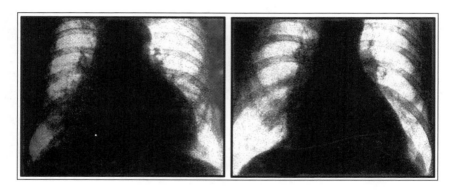

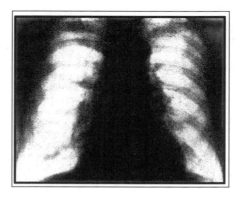

Source: Zondek H. The Myxedema Heart. *Munchen Medical WSCHR.* 1918; 65:1180.

By 1925, an article that outlined the diagnosis and treatment of heart failure associated with hypothyroidism was published in the *Journal of the American Medical Association (JAMA)*. George Fahr M.D. stated, "The shape of the heart in severe myxedema is so characteristic that Dr. Rigler, the roentgenologist (radiologist) at the hospital, diagnosed the second and third cases in my series after examination of the roentgenogram [X-ray] alone." He described this characteristic appearance as a heart, "enormously dilated in all chambers." This is one of the most common forms of CHF.[9]

The following X-rays showed the heart's dramatic return to normal size. To demonstrate that the thyroid hormones were responsible for this change, the hormones were stopped for 6 weeks. As a result, the fourth X-ray shows the heart beginning to enlarge. After the thyroid hormones were restarted, the heart size normalized once again.

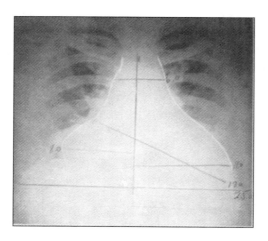

1. Frontal chest X-ray of a 46 year-old woman's heart prior to beginning thyroid. The heart is the large white mass; dark lines are shadows between the ribs. Her BMR (basal metabolic rate) was 25% below normal. Oct. 8, 1923.

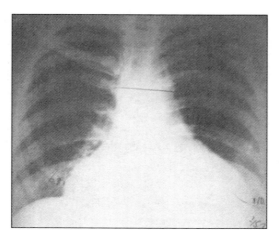

2. Twelve days after beginning thyroid medication, her BMR was 10% below normal. Oct. 24, 1923.

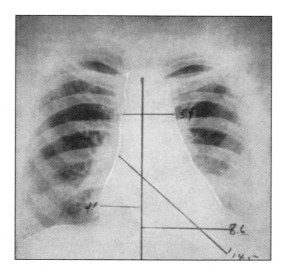

3. Sixty-eight days after beginning thyroid medication, heart returned to normal size. Her BMR was 3% above normal. Dec. 19, 1923.

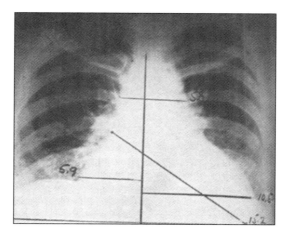

4. Six weeks after thyroid stopped, heart was enlarging again.
    Her BMR was 10% below normal. Feb. 24, 1924.

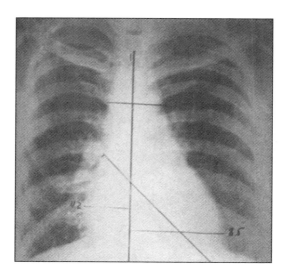

5. Five weeks after restarting thyroid, heart returned to normal
    size again. Her BMR was 5% above normal. Mar. 12, 1924.

Source: Fahr G. Myxedema Heart. *JAMA*. 1925; 84(5):345-349.
        Reprinted with permission.

Modern medical textbooks about hypothyroidism prominently mention its effect on the heart. Cardiac output (blood flow from the heart to the rest of the body) is often reduced to one half the normal value. However, most CHF patients who suffer hypothyroidism are not identified because the thyroid hormone blood tests are missing the vast majority of patients suffering from the illness. When patients are identified with hypothyroidism, the dosages that doctors have been taught to use for the last 40 years are ineffectual and do not resolve congestive heart failure.

The last medical textbook that contained "before treatment" and "after treatment" photographs was published in 1957. Its distinguished authors were Dr. Lisser, President of the American Endocrine Society, and Dr. Escamilla, both of whom spent their careers at the University of California Endocrinology Clinic in San Francisco.

The following photographs and case study are from Dr. Escamilla's and Dr. Lisser's 1957 textbook. They represent a remarkable illustration of how wrong the treatment for hypothyroidism has become.

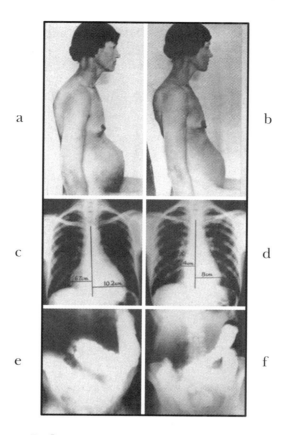

a

b

c

d

e

f

Before treatment After treatment

Source: Lisser H, and Escamilla RF. *Atlas of Clinical Endocrinology:*
Including Text of Diagnosis and Treatment. C.V. Mosby Company,
1957. Reprinted with permission.

This 45-year-old woman complained of weakness, sore and
stiff joints, slowing of mental and physical activity, impairment of
memory, slowing of speech, dryness of skin, lack of perspiration,
cold intolerance, some loss of eyebrows and body hair, increasing
constipation, and heavy periods. She also had an accumulation of
fluid in her abdominal cavity (ascites), yellowish skin (carotinemia)
an enlarged heart, and a basal metabolism rate that was 41% below

normal. The patient's appearance before and after three months of therapy demonstrates resolution of the abdominal fluid (ascites), normalization of heart size, and markedly improved tone in her colon. Her periods normalized and her heart rate increased from 51 beats per minute to 84.

The doctors named her form of hypothyroidism "internal myxedema." She did not suffer any puffiness of the skin (myxedema). Drs. Lisser and Escamilla treated her initially with 2 grains of desiccated thyroid and slowly increased the dosage to 4 grains daily. I have included this case study from their textbook to verify that these wonderful doctors prescribed 4 grains of desiccated thyroid, which enabled her complete recovery.

> After three months of proper treatment using desiccated thyroid (2 grains slowly increased to 4 grains a day), her symptoms were resolved.

For the last 40 years, endocrinologists and primary care doctors have been taught that desiccated thyroid is similar to snake oil and that a dosage of 4 grains is a massive overdose.

The Medical School Model

In the late 1980s, when I was in medical school, I saw several patients with this constellation of symptoms. Medical students were taught to remove the fluid from patients' abdomens (peritoneal cavity) with a large needle. We would prescribe medications for the heart and were instructed to use laxatives and enemas in order to relieve severe constipation.

Since I began proper treatment for hypothyroidism, none of my patients have ever developed congestive heart failure.

Unfortunately, several of my colleagues and I have found that it is extremely difficult to successfully treat patients with severe congestive heart failure. The old adage that an ounce of prevention is worth a pound of cure could not be more true.

Chapter 3
Diabetes:
Prevention and Treatment

The incidence of diabetes and its associated medical costs are staggering. It is estimated the cost of diagnosed diabetes in United States in 2012 was $245 billion. $176 billion for direct medical costs and $69 billion in reduced productivity.

According to the American Diabetes Association, 25.8 million children and adults in the United States now have diabetes, which translates into 8.3% of the population. 18.8 million have already been diagnosed and seven million people have not yet been diagnosed who are suffering from the illness.

The precursor to diabetes is called pre-diabetes and an estimated 79 million people in United States are thought to have that problem. Almost 27% of adults over age 65 suffer from diabetes. In 2004, heart disease was noted on 68% of diabetic related death certificates among people 65 years or older.

Diabetes is the leading cause of new cases of blindness. During 2005–2008, 4.2 million people with diabetes age 40 or older had diabetic retinopathy that could lead to severe vision loss. Diabetes is the leading cause of kidney failure accounting for 44% of new cases in 2008. Sixty to seventy percent of people with diabetes have mild to severe forms of nervous system damage. A majority of those with diabetes, age 20 years or older, have elevated blood pressure. In 2006, about 65,000 lower limb amputations were performed on people who suffered diabetes in America.[10]

Most people do not realize that almost all the complications that result from having diabetes are due to hardening of the arteries (arterial sclerosis or atherosclerosis). Diabetics suffer accelerated atherosclerosis identical to that associated with hypothyroidism. The complications from arterial sclerosis include blindness, kidney failure, heart attacks, gangrene, and nerve damage, as well as other complications.

What Can Be Learned
From the Historical Records?

In 1970, autopsy studies showed the rate of amputations in the non-diabetic population in Graz, Austria was five times that of the diabetic population in the United States. Antibiotics and antituberculin drugs allowed Austria's endemic hypothyroid population to survive. Hence, their overall rate of atherosclerosis was much worse than in America.[11]

Dr. Barnes eventually realized that none of his diabetic patients who had joined his study developed any additional complications.

Dr. Barnes combed the medical literature to find out if there had been any prior medical reports concerning the prevention of diabetic complications by using proper treatment for hypothyroidism. He found a study published in 1954 entitled "Coexistence of Hypothyroidism with Diabetes Mellitus" by Crosby D. Eaton M.D. The study included several hundred diabetic patients of all ages who were treated with desiccated thyroid for years. Dr. Eaton realized that the vast majority of his diabetic patients suffered hypothyroidism. He administered desiccated thyroid hormones with no adverse effect upon their diabetic condition. He reported vastly reduced incidence of complications related to diabetes, as well as the elimination of the symptoms associated with hypothyroidism.[12]

Dr. Barnes was not the first to report what now seems to be an astonishing revelation. However, he was the first doctor to backup his report with hard evidence consisting of 70,000 Graz autopsy studies, as well as his own long-term patient outcome studies. Of the 1,569 patients in Dr. Barnes study, the incidence of new cases of diabetes was quite rare. At that time, about 5% of Americans suffered from diabetes. Dr. Barnes patients had a much lower incidence of diabetes. Proper treatment for hypothyroidism greatly reduces the incidence of diabetes.

My Clinical Experience

During my 15 years of prescribing thyroid hormones, none of my patients have developed type 1 diabetes. I have treated a growing number of children and teenagers. Type 1 diabetes is the juvenile form that is life threatening and requires life-long treatment with insulin.

I have had four adult patients develop type 2 diabetes. Type 2 diabetes was formally called the adult onset form of diabetes. Unfortunately, it is increasingly being diagnosed in younger age groups. Three of these patients had not yet reached a therapeutic dosage of thyroid (more than 2 grains) when they were diagnosed with diabetes.

Only one of my patients on more than 2 grains developed type 2 diabetes. When he first came to my clinic, he was 62 years old and suffered from rheumatoid arthritis, hypothyroidism, and Hashimoto's thyroiditis. He had severe dental problems including root canals. At age 65, he developed type 2 diabetes. He still has two root canals, which pose a serious health threat. I recommend patients who have root canals read these references: *The Roots of Disease Connecting Dentistry and Medicine, Healing is Voltage, Root Canal Cover Up,* and *Let the Tooth Be Known.*[13]

Again, normal thyroid function is necessary for all the other hormone producing tissues to function normally (including the pancreas where insulin is produced).

Chapter 4
Proper Treatment for Hypothyroidism

In 1976, Dr. Barnes estimated that half of all men, women, and children in America suffered from hypothyroidism.[14]

Thyroid Stimulating Hormone (TSH) Blood Test:
Used to Diagnose and Treat Hypothyroidism

The TSH blood test was invented in the 1960s and became the "standard of care" in 1971. Currently, the normal blood test values range from 0.4 to 4.6 in America. These values have changed several times and differ in other countries. If the TSH is above 4.6, the patient is diagnosed to be hypothyroid.

If the TSH test is in the normal range, no matter how many hypothyroid symptoms people suffer, doctors are taught that their symptoms could not possibly result from hypothyroidism.

Doctors are taught that the TSH is elevated when our bodies need more thyroid hormones. If the TSH result is below normal (suppressed), doctors are taught that the patient is taking an overdose of thyroid hormones. Another reason why the TSH may be suppressed is because the patient may have <u>hyper</u>thyroidism, which is also called Graves' disease. Graves' disease occurs if the thyroid gland is producing too many thyroid hormones.

The following description and illustration should help to clarify how TSH is produced.

There are several physiological assumptions on which the validity of blood tests for hypothyroidism depends (see corresponding numbers in the following diagram):

1. The peripheral tissues transmit their need for thyroid hormones to the brain.
2. The part of the brain called the hypothalamus transmits these signals to another part of the brain called the pituitary gland.

3. The pituitary secretes TSH (thyroid stimulating hormone), which gives the signal to the thyroid gland to secrete more thyroid hormones.
4. The thyroid gland secretes thyroid hormones.
5. Thyroid hormones are transported to the peripheral tissues via the blood.

Doctors have been taught that the action of the thyroid hormones on the tissues reduces the demand for more thyroid hormones. However, recent research indicates that the pituitary has a unique enzyme that works independently from the rest of the body.

Figure 1   **Thyroid Pathways**

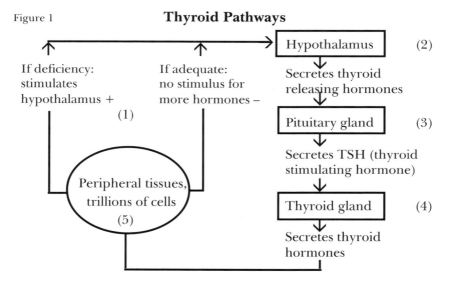

Recent Research Indicates Why the TSH Test Should No Longer Be Used for Testing and Treating Hypothyroidism

A research study was published in January 2012 by the National Academy of Hypothyroidism that provided strong evidence that the TSH blood test is not an accurate measurement of our body's thyroid function.[15]

In order to simplify this research data, I must first explain how the body utilizes thyroid hormones. There are four different forms of our own thyroid hormones. They are named T4, T3, T2, and

T1. The predominant form of thyroid secreted from our thyroid gland contains four iodine molecules and is called T4. The "T" is an amino acid named tyrosine, which is in all four forms of our thyroid. T4 is a relatively weak hormone and must be converted into T3 by an enzyme named deiodinase (de means to remove). This enzyme removes one iodine molecule and converts T4 into T3. T3 has about five times more physiological activity than T4. T2 is necessary for acute increased needs for energy. T1 has much less activity.[16]

This new research revealed that there are three different forms of deiodinases that are named D-1, D-2, and D-3. These enzymes function semi-independently.

D-1 converts T4 into T3 throughout the body but is not a significant determinant of the conversion of T4 to T3 in the pituitary. The TSH is produced in the pituitary.

D-1 is suppressed and down regulated in response to physiological and emotional stress, depression, dieting, weight gain, insulin resistance, obesity, diabetes, leptin resistance, autoimmune diseases, systemic illness, chronic fatigue, fibromyalgia, chronic pain, and exposure to toxins and plastics. In such conditions, there are reduced tissue levels of T3 everywhere in the body except the pituitary gland (which was previously unknown).

The reduced tissue levels of T3 throughout the body have previously been quoted as a beneficial response that lowers tissue metabolism. There is no evidence to justify this claim. However, there is significant evidence demonstrating a detrimental response to the lower T3 levels.

D-2 is produced by the pituitary and is regulated by intra-pituitary T3 levels. **Pituitary T3 levels usually do not correlate or provide an accurate indicator of T3 levels in the rest of the body.**

The pituitary is different from every other tissue in the body. There is a unique make up of deiodinases in the pituitary that often respond opposite to that of other tissues in the body.

Numerous conditions result in an increase in pituitary T3 while simultaneously suppressing T3 in the rest of the body. Again, these conditions are physiological and emotional stress, depression, dieting, weight gain, insulin resistance, obesity, diabetes, leptin resistance, autoimmune diseases, systemic illness, chronic fatigue, fibromyalgia, chronic pain, and exposure to toxins and plastics.

Pituitary T3 levels are determined by D-2 activity, which is 1000 times more efficient at converting T4 to T3 than the D-1 enzyme in the rest of the body and is much less sensitive to suppression by toxins and medications. In the pituitary, 80-90% of T4 is converted to T3 while only about 30-50% of T4 in the peripheral tissue is converted into active T3.

The pituitary levels of T3 are under completely different physiological control than the rest of the body. Pituitary levels of T3 will always be significantly higher than anywhere else in the body.

This research clearly shows that the TSH blood test should not be used to diagnose and treat hypothyroidism.

My Personal Experience

I was 37 years old when I completed medical school and was still in my medical residency training at age 40. At that time, my concentration began to diminish. I became cold easily. I suffered increasing joint and muscle pain and my skin became dry and itchy. My older brother and mother were already taking thyroid medication after having been diagnosed with hypothyroidism.

I sought help from my colleagues in the endocrinology department because my symptoms were characteristic of hypothyroidism. The doctors informed me that my thyroid blood tests were normal and I did not need treatment for hypothyroidism. They thought that I was working too hard and dismissed my symptoms because my TSH blood test was normal.

My chronic back pain had been worsening for many years after a high school football injury. During my last year of residency, I heard a lecture about how to treat muscle pain. I traveled to New York to study with a muscle pain specialist and planned on staying six weeks. I stayed two years before returning home to open my private practice in Missouri.

One of my teachers in New York was Dr. Hans Kraus. He was the famous pain specialist who alleviated President Kennedy's back pain using trigger point injections and exercises. Dr. Kraus worked with President Kennedy's endocrinologist, Eugene Cohen M.D. (JFK had hypothyroidism and Addison's disease). Dr. Cohen and another endocrinologist, Lawrence Sonkin M.D., Ph.D., collaborated treating each other's patients for decades. They were very much aware of the integral connection between hormonal problems, such as hypothyroidism, with chronic pain and headaches.

I told Dr. Kraus about my back pain and hypothyroid symptoms and he promptly referred me to Dr. Sonkin. After hearing my story and performing a physical exam, Dr. Sonkin placed me on thyroid hormones. I asked him about the thyroid blood tests that had prevented me from receiving treatment. Dr. Sonkin told me that the TSH blood tests were missing millions of people who had hypothyroidism.

Dr. Sonkin showed me a portion of his research. I asked why his research had not been published in a medical journal. His response was, "Because I sat in the Ivory Tower with the Mavens." Mavens are self-proclaimed experts who, in this instance, used their influence to shape the practice of medicine. The Mavens chose not to publish Dr. Sonkin's research in any endocrinology journal. Unfortunately, money, power, and ego have a profound influence on the business of medicine.

In order to help you understand Dr. Sonkin's research, I will explain a test named Basal Metabolic Rate (BMR).

Basal Metabolic Rate

Thyroid hormones control the speed and efficiency of our metabolism. Hypothyroidism slows down our metabolism. The BMR test was developed in the early 20th century to help aid doctors with the often difficult and obscure diagnosis of hypothyroidism.

The test measured a person's metabolism by monitoring oxygen consumption for a given height, weight, age, and sex. Normal values were determined from a large number of apparently healthy people. However, in order for the BMR to be accurate, the patient must be free from stress and nervous tension. Tension can result from chronic pain, neuroses, anxiety, or other problems associated with hypothyroidism.

Patients were tested after a good night sleep. They were instructed to fast after their evening meal and to travel immediately to the test location upon awakening. If they lived too far away, they were hospitalized overnight in an attempt to ensure accuracy. A tight clip was placed on their nose and a tube inserted into their mouth to measure oxygen. Stressors and tension often resulted in a normal or above average BMR despite the fact that a patient's metabolism was actually low. A British study tested 100 patients with definite hypothyroidism in 1960. The BMR test confirmed the illness in only 77 of the patients.[14]

In 1998, I recruited a Ph.D. exercise physiologist to perform basal metabolic rate testing for my pain patients. The doctor was very conscientious and tried to make certain the patients were relaxed and proper procedures followed. He performed basal metabolism tests on 50 consecutive pain patients. All of these patients had normal TSH blood tests.

My 50 patients' metabolism averaged 15% below normal. A significant number of their metabolic rates were in the 30 - 40% below normal range. Several tests were above average as well. When a basal metabolism test was previously used to aid doctors in making the diagnosis of hypothyroidism, a test result of 10% less than normal or lower was considered strongly indicative of the illness.

I sent copies of the low basal metabolic tests to the patients' primary care physicians along with my diagnosis of hypothyroidism. Almost without exception, the test results as well as the patients' textbook symptomatology were ignored. Their physicians simply felt that the TSH blood tests could not be wrong.

An unfortunate 80 year-old woman held the record low metabolism for all my patients. She initially was unable to stay awake during her office visits and summoned all her energy to travel to and from my office. The patient stated she slept for most of the previous 10 years after a new doctor stopped her thyroid medication. The doctor said her blood tests showed that she no longer needed thyroid hormones. Despite the fact she had taken the hormones for over 40 years, and was doing quite well, the thyroid hormones were stopped. Her BMR showed that her metabolic rate was 48% below normal, even though her TSH was in the normal range.

The test results from my patients and Dr. Sonkin's patients indicate that the TSH does not measure patients' metabolic rate (BMR). There are no studies in any of the medical literature showing that such a correlation exists.

Dr. Sonkin's research also illustrates how normal thyroid blood tests do not measure the BMR and are missing untold numbers of patients suffering from hypothyroidism.

Figure 2   **Therapeutic Trials (TSH and/or T4 normal)**

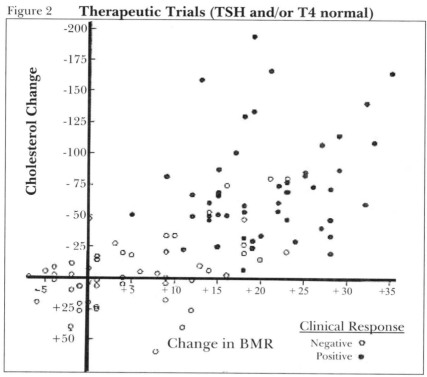

Source: Gelb H. *Clinical Management of Head, Neck, and TMJ* Pain and Dysfunction.* Philadelphia: W. B. Saunders, 1977; page 162. Reprinted with permission.

* Temporomandibular joint (TMJ) pain is another symptom of hypothyroidism.

The graph illustrates how many of Dr. Sonkin's patients with normal thyroid blood tests responded well to thyroid hormones. One hundred consecutive patients with symptoms of hypothyroidism were tested. The change in BMR and cholesterol levels were plotted on the graph. The patients represented by the darkened circles reported improvement of their symptoms. The patients represented by the clear circles reported no improvement in their symptoms (negative clinical response).

The horizontal line represents the change in BMR after a trial of thyroid hormones (a combination of T3 and T4). Two-thirds (66/100) of the patients' BMRs increased from 10% to 35%. The vertical line represents the drop in patients' cholesterol. Following treatment, over half of the patients' cholesterol dropped from 25 points to 200 points. A majority of the patients' hypothyroid symptoms improved.

The Cholesterol Connection

For the first half of the 20th century, doctors were aware that elevated cholesterol was diagnostic of hypothyroidism. In 1934, Dr. L.M. Hurxthal from the Lahey Clinic found the relation of cholesterol to the BMR was so sensitive, he suggested using serum cholesterol as a diagnostic test for hypothyroidism.[17]

Dr. Barnes checked cholesterol on all patients for 25 years. He stated, "Most younger patients and some adults may have normal or below normal cholesterol levels and still be in dire need of thyroid."[18]

My cholesterol and triglyceride levels were well within normal ranges at age 36, during my third year of medical school. Medical students practiced drawing each others' blood, while learning important lessons about blood tests. I believed my scores were normal because I excersied regularly and ate a healthful diet.

By age 41, without any change in diet or exercise, my cholesterol level had risen to 300 and my triglycerides were over 400. My symptoms of hypothyroidism had markedly worsened. Fortunately, Dr. Sonkin placed me on T4 and T3 shortly thereafter and my symptoms began to resolve. My elevated cholesterol and triglycerides normalized after 18 months of proper thyroid treatment.

I believe the most comprehensive research regarding cholesterol and the failure of statin drugs to reduce heart attacks is found in Dr. Jerry Tennant's book, *Healing is Voltage: The Handbook*.[16] I recommend his book to everyone.

24 Hour Urine T3 Test

Dr. Jacques Hertoghe, the 3rd generation Belgian endocrinologist, developed an accurate test to detect hypothyroidism. It is called the 24 hour urine T3 test and measures how much of the active form of thyroid (T3) is excreted in 24 hours. The Hertoghe method of testing and treatment is desperately needed around the world.

The following study was done by Dr. Jacques Hertoghe and two of his colleagues. Two groups of patients were treated for hypothyroidism. The first group of patients had already been diagnosed with hypothyroidism and placed on T4 by other doctors. They sought help at the clinic because the T4 treatments did not relieve their symptoms. The second group of patients had never been treated for hypothyroidism. They went to the Hertoghe clinic because they were ailing and hoped to get help for their ailments. These doctors and the senior Hertoghes had been using desiccated thyroid and treating hypothyroidism quite successfully for most of the 20th century.

In the 1970s, doctors in all the western nations were instructed to begin treating thyroid blood tests with the new synthetic T4 instead of treating patients with desiccated thyroid (that had worked quite well since the late 19th century). It did not take long for Dr. Hertoghe and his colleagues to realize that this new method of treatment was a very poor substitute for their former method, which emphasized resolution of patients' symptoms using desiccated thyroid. They stated, **"It is necessary to stress that the clinical evaluation of the patient's condition must precede interpretation of laboratory tests and not follow it."**[19]

Figure 3 highlights eight of the most common symptoms of hypothyroidism. Symptoms were measured before and after their treatment. These doctors wanted to show how well the patients' symptoms responded using treatments they had used for decades, versus the relatively new mandated treatment with synthetic thyroid.

Figure 3

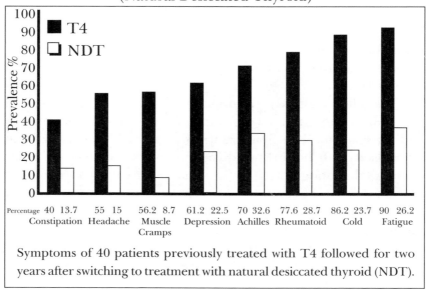

Score of Symptoms Under T4 and Under NDT
(Natural Desiccated Thyroid)

Symptoms of 40 patients previously treated with T4 followed for two years after switching to treatment with natural desiccated thyroid (NDT).

Source: Hertoghe J, Baiser WV, Eeckhaut W. Thyroid insufficiency. Is thyroxine the only valuable drug? *J Nutr Environ Med.* 2001; 11:159-166. Reprinted with permission.

The patients represented by the dark bar graph had previously been treated for hypothyroidism by other doctors. These other doctors had prescribed synthetic T4, which is one the most commonly prescribed medications in the world. Brand names of T4 include Synthroid®, Levoxyl®, levothyroxine, and Unithroid®.

Patients in the Hertoghe study who had been taking T4 were not relieved of their symptoms and sought help from the Belgian clinic. The 89 patients who had been taking T4 were switched to desiccated thyroid. Symptoms from 40 of the 89 patients were followed for about two years. The patients' symptoms markedly improved after treatment with natural desiccated thyroid (NDT).

The white bar graph represents the patients' symptoms following treatment with natural desiccated thyroid. Fatigue decreased from 90% to 26%. Cold intolerance decreased from 86% to 23%. Rheumatoid means joint and muscle pain, and was decreased from 77% to 28%. Achilles is a reflex at the back of the ankle that is often sluggish when hypothyroidism is present. Sluggish reflexes reduced from 70% to 32%. Depression decreased from 61% to 22%. Muscle cramps decreased from 56% to 8%. Headaches and migraines decreased from 55% to 15%. Constipation decreased from 40% to 13% in this group of patients.

The second page of this study includes 278 patients who had not been previously treated (see Table 5). They were also given desiccated thyroid and followed for about two years. They responded equally well.

The dosages of desiccated thyroid that were given to patients in this study ranged from 2 grains of desiccated thyroid to 5 grains. These dosages are exactly the same as the ones in Dr. Barnes' long-term study to prevent heart attacks. The average adult dosage for the T4 treated patients was 233 mg (or about 3.5 grains) and the untreated group required an average of 200 mg (about 3 grains) for most of their symptoms to resolve. Patients were followed for about two years because thyroid hormones continue to improve patients' symptoms over that length of time.

Table 5

Symptoms Score of T4 Treated Patients Who Were Subsequently Treated with Natural Desiccated Thyroid (NDT)

	Untreated		T4 Treated	
Number of patients	832	278	89	40
Symptoms score*	10.0	10.1	10.4	10.7
Urine T3 pmol	756.0	752.0	767.0	797.5
Months of treatment			38.6	33.2
Thyroxine mcg			97.6	99.7

	NDT Treated	NDT Treated
Number of patients	278	40
Symptoms score*	3.6	3.6
Urine T3 pmol	1900.0	1900.0
Months of mcg treatment	23.0	26.9
NDT mg	200.0	233.0

*The maximum possible score for symptoms was 16.
Pmol (picomol) and mcg (microgram) are units of measure.
NDT is natural desiccated thyroid.

Source: Hertoghe J, Baiser WV, Eeckhaut W. Thyroid insufficiency. Is thyroxine the only valuable drug? *J Nutr Environ Med.* 2001; 11:159-166. Reprinted with permission.

Patients in the T4 treated group had been previously diagnosed with hypothyroidism by another doctor because their TSH was elevated. When the TSH is elevated, the thyroid gland is producing very few thyroid hormones. These patients usually require a slightly higher dosage of thyroid versus the untreated group. The untreated group had not been previously diagnosed by other doctors because they had normal TSH blood tests. The untreated group required 200 mg NDT versus 233 mg in the T4 treated group.

Dr. Hertoghe and his colleagues knew that the TSH blood test was erroneous and successfully treated these patients based on their symptoms and the 24 hour urine test.

> I tell my patients that thyroid treatment is measured in months and years, not days and weeks.

My clinical experience using desiccated thyroid is quite similar to the findings in this study. These dosages are exactly what I have prescribed to restore my patients' health. The average adult dosage is 3 to 3.5 grains per day. The larger the person, the more thyroid they require to regain their health. There are always exceptions, especially if the patient's thyroid gland has been removed or destroyed by radioactive iodine, or other medications. These patients often require larger dosages.

My Clinical Experience

I began my pain clinic in 1996, and within two years I realized the vast majority of my pain patients suffered from hypothyroidism. I decided to review my pain patients' medical histories, symptoms, and physical findings after realizing the pervasiveness of hypothyroidism in my pain patients. Random chart reviews were preformed on 162 adult patients out of over 500 patients. Table 6 lists my patients' symptoms associated with hypothyroidism. There were 44 males and 118 females. Their average age was 49 years.

In Table 7, I separated 34 patients who were already being treated for hypothyroidism (with T4) out of the 162 patients.

Table 6

Starr Pain Clinic Patients: 162 Chart Reviews

	Number of Patients	Percentage
Pain	156	96
Dry Skin	137	85
Fatigue	134	83
Brittle/Ridged Nails	131	81
Menstrual problems (females)	81	69
Depression	91	57
Myxedema:		
Moderate to Marked	88	54
Cold Intolerance	86	53
Insomnia	86	53
Delayed Ankle Reflexes	80	49
Hysterectomy (females)	48	41
Allergies	66	41
Cold Hands or Feet	62	38
Weight Gain	61	38
Constipation	52	32
High Blood Pressure	50	31
Tension (anxiety)	47	29
Headaches	46	28
Hair Loss	45	28
TMJ - Teeth Clenching	40	25
Paresthesias (tingling)	38	24
Hypothyroidism, Type 1	34	21
Tremor	31	19
Heart Disease	27	17
Diabetes	26	16
Heat Intolerance	25	15
Cancer	15	9
Autoimmune Disease	12	7
Hypoglycemia	11	7
Emphysema	8	5

Table 7   **Starr Pain Clinic Patients with**
Prior Diagnosis of Hypothyroidism

	Number of Patients	Percentage
Already receiving treatment (T4, i.e. levothyroxine), dosage range 0.1 mg (100 mcg) to 0.2 mg (200 mcg) per day.		
Hypothyroidism Type 1	34	100
Dry Skin	29	85
Fatigue	29	85
Brittle/Ridged Nails	28	82
Menstrual Problems (females)	20	67
Cold Intolerance	22	65
Depression	20	59
Myxedema:		
Moderate to Marked	19	56
Delayed Ankle Reflexes	19	56
Cold Hands or Feet	17	50
Insomnia	17	50
Hair Loss	16	47
Allergies	15	44
Tension (anxiety)	14	41
Weight Gain	14	41
High Blood Pressure	10	29
Hysterectomy (females)	7	23
Diabetes	9	26
Heat Intolerance	9	26
Paresthesias (tingling)	9	26
Tremor	7	21
Constipation	7	21
TMJ - Teeth Clenching	7	21
Headaches	6	18
Heart Disease	5	15
Cancer	4	12
Emphysema	3	9

Patients in Table 7, who were already being treated for hypothyroidism with T4, suffered just as many symptoms related to the illness as those who had not begun any treatment for hypothyroidism in Table 6.

Again, my findings agree with those from the Hertoghe study. Obviously, treatment using T4 is woefully lacking. Many of these patients' symptoms resolved after additional thyroid hormones were given.

I refer all inquiries that my office receives from Europe to the Belgian clinic:

Thierry Hertoghe
Brussels, Belgium
+ 32 2 736 68 68
www.hertoghe.eu
thhertoghe@gmx.net

Therese Hertoghe
Internal Medicine
Rue Pierre Delacroix, 23
1150 Brussels
00 32 2 463 03 00

Dr. Jacques Hertoghe and his colleagues introduced the T3 24 hour urine test in 1984. This test has proven itself to be the only reliable laboratory method that accurately measures thyroid function. Dr. Barnes' basal temperature test is the next best measure. Jerry Tennant M.D. has pioneered another method using blood tests that may prove to be effective as well.[20]

Basal Temperature

Dr. Barnes measured the BMR as well as the basal temperature on every patient he treated. Numerous doctors had previously reported that a low basal temperature was almost always found in those suffering from hypothyroidism.[21] During a tour of duty in World War II, Dr. Barnes studied 1,000 soldiers' temperatures. Prior to reveille, one thermometer would be placed in their mouth, one in their arm pit (axilla), and one in their rectum. If no sign of upper respiratory infection was present, he found that the oral temperature was within one tenth degree of the axillary temperature. The rectal temperature was eight tenths higher.

These findings conflict with standard medical textbooks that state the axillary temperature is one degree Fahrenheit lower than the oral temperature and two degrees Fahrenheit below the rectal temperature. However, no references are given to support their findings. Thyroid textbooks almost all state that the basal temperature test is invalid. Once again, absolutely no references are given. Dr. Barnes published his findings in his article entitled "Basal Temperature versus Basal Metabolism", which was published in the *Journal of the American Medical Association (JAMA)* in 1942.[22]

After understanding Dr. Barnes research, I have utilized the basal temperature in all of the patients that I have treated for hypothyroidism. Hypothyroid patients' temperatures are almost always below normal before they begin treatment. There are rare exceptions.

One of my former patients suffered emphysema. Her basal temperature was above normal because she had chronic lung infections, which are almost always present in emphysema patients. She had marked myxedema, a low hoarse voice, chronic pain, and anxiety. She also was over six feet tall. Many of her symptoms resolved after her dosage was slowly raised to 4 grains.

Just like the BMR, the basal temperature should be taken after a good night rest with no food, exercise, or excitement for 12 hours. Many patients who are hypothyroid may cover themselves with an excess number of blankets or quilts, sleep on a heated waterbed, wear long underwear, or layers of clothes to bed. All of these measures will falsely elevate the basal temperature. Women's temperatures fluctuate during their menstrual cycle, and their tests should be taken on the second and third days after menstrual flow starts. Babies and small children may be checked by rectal temperature for two minutes. I recommend a Geratherm thermometer.

To test your basal temperature, the thermometer is placed snugly in the armpit for 10 minutes before arising in the morning. Dr. Barnes found that temperature readings of 97.8 to 98.2° Fahrenheit (36.6 to 36.8° Celsius) were normal. Normal rectal temperatures are eight tenths degree higher, 98.6 to 99.2° Fahrenheit (37 to 37.3° Celsius).

During his lectures, Dr. Barnes stated that many of the adult patients he treated never attained normal basal body temperatures, even though they were given all the thyroid they were able to tolerate. Many of my adult patients' temperatures remain below normal even though their symptoms resolve.

The most important temperature readings are prior to being diagnosed with hypothyroidism. Once the diagnosis of hypothyroidism has been established and patients begin taking thyroid hormones, their basal temperatures will fluctuate for many months. The patients' temperatures will gradually increase as the thyroid dosage is raised.

My Recommendations About How to Begin Treatment for Hypothyroidism

> A note of caution: Thyroid hormones are among the most powerful medications known to man.

Cardiac output (blood flow to the body from the heart) is often significantly decreased due to hypothyroidism. When beginning even small dosages of thyroid hormones, the heart muscle becomes stronger and beats more forcefully. If the coronary arteries supplying the heart are compromised by arterial sclerosis, the arteries may not be able to accommodate the increased blood flow, which is required. When the heart is deprived of the necessary blood flow, a heart attack may occur. Please follow my recommendations closely in order to minimize this danger.

Rule#1: Patients who have suffered a heart attack should not begin any thyroid medication for two months following a heart attack. I recommend such patients begin nitric oxide (NEO-40 www.neogenis.com) two or three times daily to help their arteries and heart begin to recover. NEO-40 may be started immediately following a heart attack.

After 60 days, I recommend beginning 0.25 grains of thyroid every other day and slowly increasing the dosage by 0.25 grains every six or eight weeks until reaching a maximum of 2 grains daily. Dr. Barnes stated that anyone who has had a heart attack is much more sensitive to thyroid medication and should never take more than 2 grains of thyroid daily. My clinical experience is in complete agreement with Dr. Barnes' findings. However, almost every heart attack patient will require 2 grains of desiccated thyroid or the equivalent dosage of T4 and T3 if they have Hashimoto's (T4-76 mcg and T3-18 mcg).

Four of my patients suffered heart attacks within several months of beginning treatment with desiccated thyroid. I believe it is extremely prudent to begin thyroid hormones very slowly in anyone suspected of having coronary artery disease. Older patients who have had chronic dental problems and long-term hypothyroidism are at risk, especially if there is a family history of heart attack.

Rule #2: Patients who have high blood pressure must also begin thyroid medication cautiously. Too much thyroid medication initially will often further elevate their blood pressure and may cause serious problems. Begin 0.25 grains daily and increase the dosage by the same amount every six or eight weeks. If the blood pressure elevates, increase the dosage more gradually. Have the patients monitor their blood pressure at least twice a week and instruct them to stop their thyroid and report to their doctor if their pressure increases.

As they reach therapeutic levels of thyroid, their blood pressure often begins to drop. It may take one or two years for some patients to respond. Slowly wean patients off their blood pressure medications as pressure drops. It is often dangerous to stop blood pressure medications abruptly.

People who have advanced arterial disease may never be able to lower their blood pressure. Dr. Barnes reported such patients lived longer by taking thyroid versus similar patients who were not on thyroid.

Rule #3: A red flag for mild adrenal deficiency, iodine deficiency, thyroid antibodies, or environmental toxicity is a worsening of hypothyroid symptoms as the dosage is gradually increased. Stop or decrease the dosage of thyroid and address these problems should they occur. Less fatigue and symptomatic relief is the expected response.

If the basal temperature begins to decline, in addition to worsening symptoms, adrenal deficiency is almost always to blame. My first book includes chapters about adrenal deficiency, Hashimoto's, and Graves' disease.

Rule #4: There are always exceptions. Some patients have great difficulty tolerating any T4 and T3 preparations, including desiccated thyroid. My first book includes detailed recommendations for even the most difficult patients.[23]

General Recommendations

After doctors discovered how to successfully treat hypothyroidism in the late 1800s, there were no diagnostic tests to help them determine whether or not a patient suffered from hypothyroidism. Patients' medical histories, symptoms, and physical findings, combined with their doctors' awareness were the only means for making the diagnosis. A trial of thyroid hormones, leading to the resolution of the patient's symptoms and physical manifestations, was confirmation of a correct diagnosis. When combined with basal temperatures, I believe this method of treatment remains a viable option.

People who have below normal basal temperatures and suffer symptoms that are associated with hypothyroidism should begin a trial of thyroid hormones. Others with low basal temperatures and a family history that includes illnesses resulting from hypothyroidism, such as heart attacks or diabetes, should also begin a trial of thyroid hormones.

For most patients, I recommend 0.25 grains first thing in the morning on an empty stomach. Wait 30 minutes before eating because minerals block the absorption of the hormones. Increase the dosage monthly for adults. Younger patients who are relatively healthy may begin 0.5 grains and increase 0.5 grains monthly.

Estrogens protect the arteries of women who continue to have menstrual cycles. If these women do not have severe allergies or Hashimoto's disease, they may also increase their dosage by 0.5 grains every month.

As previously stated, the average adult dosage is about 3 grains every day. Dr. Barnes stated, "The bigger the beast, the bigger the bigger the bullet!" I have treated several 300 pound patients with 5 or 6 grains a day.

There are occasional patients who do not tolerate T3. Dr. Sonkin treated one family very successfully using large dosages of Synthroid (T4). A woman required 3 mg (about 30 times the amount that doctors currently recommend) and her son required 2.7 mg for restoration of their health. I asked Dr. Sonkin how he could possibly prescribe so much thyroid medication. His response was, "Because it took that much to wake them up!" The patients demonstrated no side effects and their symptoms markedly improved. Dr. Sonkin gradually increased their dosages and noted that the son had shown symptoms of thyrotoxicosis (an overdose) at 2.9 mg, which necessitated the slight decrease to 2.7 mg.[24]

Treating Children and Teens

Small children may begin 0.25 grains every other day. Compounding pharmacies can make liquid preparations for small children. I increase the dosage of thyroid every two months when treating children. Almost all the children that I have treated attained normal basal temperatures when they reached their correct dosage of thyroid. As they grow, their temperatures decline and their dosages are gradually increased. I insist that the parents monitor their child's heart rate and basal temperature every few weeks. The normal heart rate is much faster in children than adult heart rates and these rates are easily found on the Internet.

If a child's basal temperature is raised above normal, after beginning thyroid, immediately stop the thyroid until the temperature returns to the normal range. Begin a lower dosage of thyroid. Hyperthermia (elevated basal temperature above normal) indicates <u>hyper</u>thyroidism and can cause severe problems including death. Of course, this does not apply if the child is ill and has a fever.

A heart rate above normal (when resting) is a strong indication that the patient is not tolerating the thyroid hormones. Additional symptoms of intolerance include palpitations, shortness of breath, chest pain, increased fatigue, increased anxiety, increased insomnia, trembling hands, and increased joint and muscle pain.

Many of the teenagers I have treated eventually required between 2 and 3 grains a day, depending upon their size. Many teens are the size of adults and require similar dosages.

Treatment for Hashimoto's and Graves' Disease

The incidence of autoimmune thyroid disease called Hashimoto's thyroiditis is rapidly increasing in America. Hashimoto's disease means your immune system is attacking your own thyroid gland. A recent study indicated that about 5% of Americans may be affected.[25]

None of Dr. Barnes' four books mentioned Hashimoto's thyroiditis. It was very rare at that time. Near the end of his recorded lecture, Dr. Barnes answered questions from the doctors who were in attendance. When asked about Hashimoto's, Dr. Barnes stated that you must use the synthetic hormones if the patent has Hashimoto's.[11]

The synthetic hormones are levothyroxine or L-thyroxin (T4) and Triiodothyronine (T3). The generic name for T3 is liothyronine and the brand name is Cytomel®.

Why would Dr. Barnes recommend synthetic hormones? Desiccated porcine (pig) thyroid is almost identical to our own thyroid gland. Pigs are genetically quite similar to humans. If the body is attacking the thyroid gland, adding more glandular thyroid is like adding fuel to the fire. However, there are a small number of patients who feel much better when taking desiccated thyroid, in spite of the fact that they have Hashimoto's disease.

The tests to determine if you have Hashimoto's are called tissue peroxidase antibodies (TPO antibodies) and thyroglobulin antibodies. If you are found to have Hashimoto's and your basal temperature is below normal, I recommend taking a combination of T4 and T3 thyroid hormones.

Hashimoto's and non-Hashimoto's patients require similar dosages; adults and children alike.

Almost all of my patients who have had Graves' disease have already had chemical destruction or surgical removal of their thyroid glands. Patients with a history of Graves' usually require synthetic T4 and T3 in order to restore their health.

A new book authored by Mary Shomon entitled *Living Well With Graves' Disease and Hyperthyroidism* offers more conservative treatments to reverse Graves' disease. Additional information is available on a growing number of Web sites including aboutthyroid. com, stopthethyroidmadness.com, and brodabarnes.org.

I always check for thyroid antibodies after chemical destruction or removal of the thyroid gland. In spite of the fact that the thyroid gland has been destroyed or removed, patients with a history of autoimmune thyroid illnesses often have high levels of thyroid antibodies.

Depending upon whether or not patients have thyroid antibodies usually dictates whether they will require T4 and T3 versus desiccated thyroid. I have had two average-sized adult patients who required 6 grains of thyroid to feel well after removal of their thyroid gland. I gradually increased their dosages over many months.

Patients who have autoimmune thyroid illnesses often suffer from severe allergies. I recommend that these patients seek help from environmental medicine physicians. Doctors belonging to the American Academy of Environmental Medicine (aaem. com) are able to diagnose and successfully treat severe food and environmental allergies much more effectively than other allergists.

Conversion Ratios of Thyroid Hormones

Desiccated thyroid contains glandular thyroid and is measured in milligrams. One grain of desiccated thyroid weighs about 65 mg and contains 38 micrograms of T4 and 9 micrograms of T3. Armour thyroid dosages are slightly different because they reference 1 grain = 60 mg. However, the stated amounts of T4 and T3 are the same (T4-38 mcg and T3-9 mcg).

Synthetic T4 and T3 are bio-identical synthetic hormones that are derived from sugar beets. T4 and T3 are measured in micrograms.

Pharmacies must use fillers to accurately measure microgram dosages. Many of my patients who had autoimmune thyroid illnesses became allergic to the most common filler, which is named methylcellulose. It is derived from pine and is allergenic. I recommend using potato starch, acidophilus, or Avicel® for fillers because they less allergenic. I have found that calcium carbonate also works well, in spite of the fact that calcium is supposed to block absorption of thyroid hormones.

Conversion of grains to desiccated thyroid:

     1 grain = T4-38 mcg and T3-9 mcg

  0.25 grains = T4-9.5 mcg and T3-2.25 mcg
     2 grains = T4-76 mcg and T3-18 mcg
     3 grains = T4-114 mcg and T3-27 mcg.

A number of countries, including Brazil, have never had access to desiccated thyroid. A doctor from Brazil is a patient of mine. He read my first book and came to my clinic in Arizona. His health has improved since he began desiccated thyroid.

TOXIC SOUP
Umbilical Cord Blood Study

A 2004 U.S. study by the Environmental Working Group (EWG) revealed that pregnant women's umbilical cord blood is contaminated with an average of 200 industrial chemicals and pollutants. Of the 287 chemicals detected, 180 are known to cause cancer in humans or animals, 217 are toxic to the brain and nervous system, and 208 cause birth defects or abnormal development in animals.

In 2009, EWG repeated the study and found an average of 232 chemicals in umbilical cord blood.[26]

If you do the math, most of these toxins cause all three problems. These are noxious poisons.

What we do to our planet, we do to ourselves.

In addition to being poisonous, a majority of these toxins adversely affect most of our hormones including the thyroid. A wonderful book on this subject is *Our Stolen Future*. The Web site (ourstolenfuture.org) is a great resource about how to protect yourself and your children from toxins that are adversely affecting our hormones. Appendix B lists the Mechanisms of Thyroid Hormone Disruption by Synthetic Chemicals.

If you have any of the conditions listed throughout this book, you should seek help from a physician who understands how to properly diagnose and treat hypothyroidism.

Chapter 5
Conclusion

The following quote is from Dr. Lisser's and Dr. Escamilla's textbook regarding adult hypothyroidism:

"Most characteristic are the dramatic benefits from treatment with desiccated thyroid, which effects reversal of most of the abnormalities to or toward normal. Milder instances are far more common and frequently go unrecognized, but likewise are helped materially by proper replacement therapy. A suspicious alertness to this diagnosis is desirable and should be followed by laboratory corroboration; confirmation by a therapeutic trial of thyroid substance is justifiable."[27]

Drs. Lisser and Escamilla are telling us that when the symptoms of hypothyroidism are present, a trial of thyroid hormones is justified.

Unfortunately, for the last 40 years, the test to confirm the diagnosis is erroneous. As a result, doctors no longer give therapeutic trials of thyroid hormones, especially desiccated thyroid.

TSH Tests Mandated

Doctors in all western nations are mandated by their licensing boards (who control of their medical licenses) to treat hypothyroid patients based upon their TSH test results. Doctors are generally forced to use the synthetic T4 to treat patients. Additionally, all formal medical training for the last 40 years has instructed doctors to prescribe T4.

During my lectures in Sweden, I learned that Swedish doctors were required to base treatment for their hypothyroid patients upon the TSH blood tests. They were also directed to use synthetic T4. The Swedish branch of government that controls prescription drugs is called the Läkemedelsverket. Swedish doctors must apply for a special license in order to treat their patients with desiccated thyroid. Unfortunately, such applications are rarely granted.

As previously stated, when taking more than 2 grains of thyroid per day, the TSH blood tests will almost always indicate that patients are on too much thyroid. This results in a reduction of their dosage. Therefore, they will never be able to achieve a therapeutic dosage that would eliminate their symptoms and prevent heart attacks, congestive heart failure, and diabetes.

A Canadian doctor, who is a friend of mine, was sanctioned by the Canadian medical board. He had been treating his patients with desiccated thyroid and was prescribing large enough dosages to resolve his patients' symptoms. The Canadian medical board now monitors his treatments to make certain that he follows the TSH mandate.

Several years ago at an alternative medical conference, it was announced that the number one reason doctors lose their medical licenses in America was due to their usage of desiccated thyroid, and not basing their treatment on the TSH blood test. In addition, some insurance companies refuse to pay doctors for their treatments if they do not use synthetic T4 and follow the TSH mandate.

The American way has now become one with the global corporate rat race to accumulate as much money as possible. I do not believe that it is an exaggeration to state that untold billions of people are suffering as a result. For many decades, research studies at university hospitals have been funded by pharmaceutical companies and large corporations. Both entities are reaping huge profits and place all their efforts on maintaining the status quo. This has significantly influenced the way medicine has been practiced.

Chapter 6
IT IS TIME TO TAKE BACK OUR FREEDOM

Newsweek magazine published a cover story on February 8, 2010 about the efficacy of antidepressant drugs entitled "The Depressing News about Antidepressants." A Freedom of Information Act was required to force the FDA to release all of the research studies about whether or not antidepressant drugs actually worked to resolve depression. It turned out that the FDA had released only the research showing beneficial responses. The FDA had held back almost all of the studies that showed a number of these medications were no more effective than placebos.[28]

One example of a harmful product being released for consumer usage was when the FDA granted approval for aspartame, an artificial sweetener. Scientists had already proven that aspartame breaks down into methanol (wood alcohol). Our bodies' convert methanol into formaldehyde. Formaldehyde is a potent toxin and proven carcinogen. Additional information, is available online.[29]

Another example concerns the drug Vioxx®. It is a pain killer that resulted in as many as 55,000 premature deaths from heart attacks and strokes. More information is available on the Internet:

www.ucsusa.org/scientific_integrity/abuses_of_science/vioxx.html

Fukushima – Impending Disaster?
The ongoing radiation leak from the Fukushima Daiichi nuclear power plant is a disaster in progress. Radiation continues to leak from the three reactors that melted down. In order to understand what we may expect to occur from this disaster, a large body of information already exists regarding the Chernobyl nuclear power plant meltdown that occurred in 1986.

The incidence of thyroid cancers around Chernobyl far exceeded initial estimates. In addition, the forms of thyroid cancer were more aggressive than expected. The following graph shows the expected rate of thyroid cancers versus those that occurred. Physicians should review the 327 page report from the *Annals of the New York Academy of Sciences*. It represents over 20 years of tracking the actual medical consequences from the Chernobyl disaster. The full report is available at:

Chernobyl: Consequences of the Catastrophe for People and the Environment. *Ann N Y Acad Sci.* 2009; 1181(viixiii):1-327. Available on the Internet at: www.nyas.org/publications/annals/Detail.aspx?cid=f3f3bd16-51ba-4d7b-a086-753f44b3bfc1. Accessed January 14, 2014.

Figure 4   **Thyroid Cancers Resulting from the Chernobyl Disaster**

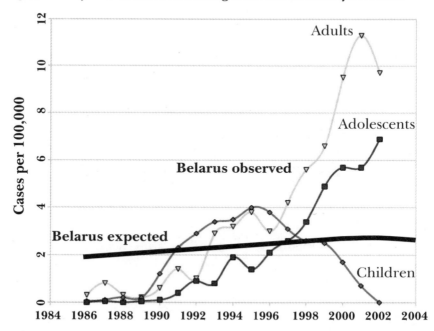

Figure 4. Expected thyroid cancers versus actual cases for children, adolescents, and adults in Belarus.

Sources: Wikipedia Web site. Chernobyl disaster. Available at: en.wikipedia.org/wiki/Chernobyl_disaster. Accessed January 14, 2014. Photo Wikimedia commons.

Malko MV. Assessment of Chernobyl Medical Consequences Accident. In Bloko I, Sandownichik T, Labunska I, Vlkov I, (Eds). The effects on the Human victims of the Chernobyl catastrophe. *Greenpeace International, Amsterdam.* 2007; pages 194-245.

Fallout In the United States from Nuclear Testing

Below is an example of how the government did not protect our populace from ongoing radiation exposure. Americans were not informed about the dangers from radiation during the above ground nuclear tests that took place from 1951-1962. No precautions were given to our citizens and the government did not make a concerted effort to track the deleterious health effects that may have resulted.

Figure 5 Radiation Exposure from Nuclear Testing 1951-1962

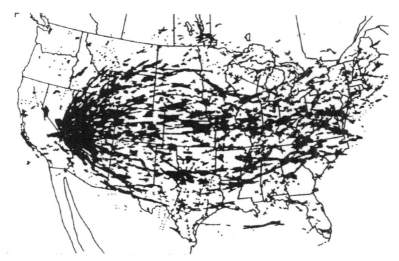

Source: Miller R. *Under the Cloud: The Decades of Nuclear Testing.* Two Sixty Press, 1999. Reprinted with permission.

My brother, Steven Starr, is one of the foremost experts regarding all things nuclear. He is a International Consultant/Educator for Nuclear Disarmament (USA); Associate member, Nuclear Age Peace Foundation (USA); Senior Scientist, Physicians for Social Responsibility; and Director of Clinical Laboratory Science Program at the University of Missouri-Columbia. The following links were recommended by Steven:

www.nucleardarkness.org
www.ratical.org/radiation/Fukushima/StevenStarr.html
www.fairewinds.org

Steven works with Helen Caldicott, M.D., who is a world renowned nuclear expert and has written several books that I recommend. She also has a number of interviews on the Internet:

www.helencaldicott.com/
www.youtube.com/watch?v=3GW1-HnvAfM

I learned recently that the majority of Americans are in favor of voting all of the current members of our Congress and Senate out of office in order to have a fresh start. I am also in favor of replacing most of the bureaucrats in the FDA and installing independent scientific leadership.

I hope and pray that all will agree to vote for REAL change!

You can fool all the people some of the time, and some of the people all the time, but you cannot fool all the people all the time.

– Abraham Lincoln (1809-1865)

America will never be destroyed from the outside. If we falter and lose our freedoms, it will be because we destroyed ourselves.

– Abraham Lincoln (1809-1865)

Appendix A
Physiologic Functions of the Thyroid Hormones

Source: Guyton A. *Textbook of Medical Physiology*. Philadelphia: WB Saunders Company, 2000. Pages 934-938. Reprinted with permission from Elsevier.

Thyroid Hormones Increase the Transcription of Large Numbers of Genes

The general effect of thyroid hormone is to activate nuclear transcription of large numbers of genes. Therefore, in virtually all cells of the body, great numbers of proteins, and other substances are synthesized. The net result is generalized increase in functional activity throughout the body.

Most of the thyroxine secreted by the thyroid is converted to triiodothyronine. Before acting on the genes to increase genetic transcription, one iodide is removed from almost all the thyroxine, thus forming triiodothyronine. Intracellular thyroid hormone receptors have a very high affinity for triiodothyronine. Consequently, about 90% of the thyroid hormone molecules that bind with the receptors is triiodothyronine and only 10% thyroxine.

Thyroid hormones activate nuclear receptors. The thyroid receptors are either attached to the DNA genetic strands or located in proximity to them. On binding with thyroid hormone, the receptors become activated and initiate the transcription process. Then large numbers of different types of messenger RNA are formed, followed within another few minutes or hours by RNA translation on the cytoplasmic ribosomes to form hundreds of new intracellular proteins. However, not all the proteins are increased by similar percentages — some only slightly and others at least as much as six-fold. It is believed that most, if not all, of the actions of thyroid hormone result from the subsequent enzymatic and other functions of these new proteins.

Thyroid Hormones Increase Cellular Metabolic Activity

The thyroid hormones increase the metabolic activities of almost all the tissues of the body. The basal metabolic rate can increase from 60% to 100% above normal when large quantities of the hormones are secreted. The rate of utilization of foods for energy is greatly accelerated. Although the rate of protein synthesis is increased, at the same time the rate of protein catabolism is also increased. The growth rate of young people is greatly accelerated. The mental processes are excited, and the activities of most of the other endocrine glands are increased.

Thyroid hormones increase the number and activity of mito-chondria. When thyroxine or triiodothyronine is given to an animal, the mitochondria in most cells of the animal's body increase in size as well as number. Furthermore, the total membrane surface area of the mitochondria increases almost directly in proportion to the increased metabolic rate of the whole animal. Therefore, one of principle functions of thyroxine might be simply to increase the number and activity of mitochondria, which in turn increases the rate of formation of adenosine triphosphate (ATP) to energize cellular function. However, the increase in the number and activity of mitochondria could be the result of increased activity of the cells, as well as the cause of the increase.

Thyroid hormones increase active transport of ions through cell membranes. One of the enzymes that becomes increased in response to thyroid hormone is Na, K-ATPase. This in turn increases the rate of transport of both sodium and potassium ions through the cell membranes of some tissue. Because this process uses energy and increases the amount of heat produced in the body, it has been suggested that this might be one of the mechanisms by which thyroid hormone increases the body's metabolic rate. In fact, thyroid hormone also causes the cell membranes of most cells to become leaky to sodium ions, which further activates the sodium pump and further increases heat production.

Effect of Thyroid Hormone on Growth
Thyroid hormone has both general and specific effects on growth. For instance, it has long been known that thyroid hormone is essential for the metamorphic change of the tadpole into the frog.

In humans, the effect of thyroid hormone on growth is manifest mainly in growing children. In those who are hypothyroid, the rate of growth is greatly retarded. In those who are hypothyroid, excessive skeletal growth often occurs, causing the child to become considerably taller at an earlier age. However, the bones also mature more rapidly and the epiphyses close at an early age, so that the duration of growth and the eventual height of the adult may actually be shortened.

An important effect of thyroid hormone is to promote growth and development of the brain during fetal life and for the first few years of postnatal life. If the fetus does not secrete sufficient quantities of thyroid hormone, growth and maturation of the brain both before birth and afterward are greatly retarded, and the brain remains smaller than normal. Without specific thyroid therapy within days or weeks after birth the child without a thyroid gland will remain mentally deficient throughout life.

Effect of Thyroid Hormone on Specific Bodily Mechanisms

Stimulation of Carbohydrates Metabolism. Thyroid hormone stimulates almost all aspects of carbohydrate metabolism, including rapid uptake of glucose by the cells, enhanced glycolysis, enhanced gluconeogenesis, increased rate of absorption from the gastrointestinal tract, and even increased insulin secretion with its resultant secondary effects on carbohydrate metabolism. All these effects probably result from the overall increase in cellular metabolic enzymes caused by thyroid hormone.

Stimulation of Fat Metabolism. Essentially all aspects of fat metabolism are also enhanced under the influence of thyroid hormone. In particular, lipids are mobilized rapidly from the fat tissue, which decreases the fat stores of the body to a greater extent than almost any other tissue element. This also increases the free fatty acid concentration in the plasma and greatly accelerates the oxidation of free fatty acids by the cells.

Effect on plasma and liver fats. Increased thyroid hormone decreases the concentrations of cholesterol, phospholipids, and triglycerides in the plasma, even though it increases the free fatty acids. Conversely, decreased thyroid secretion greatly increases the plasma concentrations of cholesterol, phospholipids, and triglycerides and almost always causes excessive deposition of fat in the liver as well. The large increase in circulation plasma cholesterol in prolonged hypothyroidism is often associated with severe arteriosclerosis.

One of the mechanisms by which thyroid hormone decreases the plasma cholesterol concentration is to increase significantly the rate of cholesterol secretion in the bile and consequent loss in the feces. A possible mechanism for the increased cholesterol secretion is that thyroid hormone induces increased numbers of low-density lipoprotein receptors on the liver cells, leading to rapid removal of low-density lipoproteins from the plasma by the liver and subsequent secretion of cholesterol in these lipoproteins by the liver cells.

Increased Requirement for Vitamins. Because thyroid hormone increases the quantities of many bodily enzymes and because vitamins are essential parts of some of the enzymes or coenzymes, thyroid hormone causes increased need for vitamins. Therefore, a relative vitamin deficiency can occur when excess thyroid hormone is secreted, unless at the same time increased quantities of vitamins are made available.

Increased Basal Metabolic Rate. Because thyroid hormone increases metabolism in almost all cells of the body, excessive quantities of the hormone can occasionally increase the basal metabolic rate from 60% to 100% above normal. Conversely, when no thyroid hormone is produced, the basal metabolic rate falls to almost one-half normal. Extreme amounts of the hormones are required to cause very high basal metabolic rates.

Decreased Body Weight. Greatly increased thyroid hormone almost always decreases the body weight, and greatly decreased hormone almost always increases body weight; these effects do not always occur, because thyroid hormone also increases the appetite, and this may counterbalance the change in the metabolic rate.

Effect of Thyroid Hormones on the Cardiovascular System

Increased Blood Flow and Cardiac Output. Increased metabolism in the tissues causes more rapid utilization of oxygen than normal and release of greater than normal quantities of metabolic end products from the tissues. These effects cause vasodilatation in most body tissues, thus increasing blood flow in the skin because of the increased need for heat elimination from the body.

As a consequence of the increased blood flow, cardiac output also increases, sometimes rising to 60% or more above normal when excessive thyroid hormone is present and falling to only 50% of normal in very severe hypothyroidism.

Increased Heart Rate. The heart rate increases considerably more under the influence of thyroid hormone than would be expected from the increase in cardiac output. Therefore, thyroid hormone seems to have a direct effect on the excitability of the heart, which in turn increases the heart rate. This rate is one of the sensitive physical signs that the clinician uses in determining whether a patient has excessive or diminished thyroid hormone production.

Increased Heart Strength. The increased enzymatic activity caused by thyroid hormone production apparently increases the strength of the heart when only a slight excess of thyroid hormone is secreted. This is analogous to the marked increase in the heart muscle strength that occurs in mild fevers and during exercise. However, when thyroid hormone is increased markedly, the heart muscle strength becomes depressed because of long-term excessive protein catabolism. Indeed, some severely thyrotoxic patients die of cardiac decompensation secondary to myocardial failure and to increased cardiac load imposed by the increase in cardiac output.

Normal Arterial Pressure. The mean arterial pressure usually remains about normal after administration of thyroid hormone. However, because of increased blood flow through the tissues between heartbeats, the pulse pressure is often increased, with the systolic pressure elevated in <u>hyper</u>thyroidism 10 to 15 mm Hg and the diastolic pressure reduced a corresponding amount.

Increased Respiration. The increased rate of metabolism increases the utilization of oxygen and formation of carbon dioxide; these effects activate all the mechanisms that increase the rate and depth of respiration.

Increased Gastrointestinal Motility. In addition to increased appetite and food intake, which had been discussed, thyroid hormone increases both the rates of secretion of the digestive juices and the motility of the gastrointestinal tract. Diarrhea often results from <u>hyper</u>thyroidism. Lack of thyroid hormone can cause constipation.

Excitatory Effects on the Central Nervous System. In general, thyroid hormone increases the rapidity of cerebration but also often dissociates this; conversely, lack of thyroid hormone decreases this function. The <u>hyper</u>thyroid individual is likely to have extreme nervousness and many psychoneurotic tendencies, such as anxiety complexes, extreme worry, and paranoia.

Effect on the Function of the Muscles. Slight increase in thyroid hormone usually makes the muscles react with vigor, but when the quantity of hormone becomes excessive, the muscles become weakened because of excess protein catabolism. Conversely, lack of thyroid hormone causes the muscles to become sluggish, and they relax slowly after contraction.

Muscle Tremor. One of the most characteristic signs of <u>hyper</u>thyroidism is a fine muscle tremor. This is not the coarse tremor that occurs in Parkinson's disease or in shivering, because it occurs at the rapid frequency of 10 to 15 times per second. The tremor can be observed easily by placing a sheet of paper on the extended fingers and noting the degree of vibration of the paper. This tremor is believed to be caused by increased reactivity of the neuronal synapses in the areas of the spinal cord that control muscle tone. The tremor is an important means for assessing the degree of thyroid hormone effect on the central nervous system.

Effect on Sleep. Because of the exhausting effect of thyroid hormone on the musculature and on the central nervous system, the hyperthyroid subject often has a feeling of constant tiredness; but because of the excitable effects of thyroid hormone on the synapses, it is difficult to sleep. Conversely, extreme somnolence is characteristic of hypothyroidism, with sleep sometimes lasting 12 to 14 hours a day.

Effect on Other Endocrine Glands. Increased thyroid hormone increases the rates of secretion of most other endocrine glands, but it also increases the need of the tissues for the hormones. For instance, increased thyroxine secretion increases the rate of glucose metabolism everywhere in the body, and therefore, causes a corresponding need for increased insulin secretion by the pancreas. Also, thyroid hormone increases many metabolic activities related to bone formation and, as a consequence, increases the need for parathyroid hormone. Finally, thyroid hormone increases the rate at which adrenal glucocorticoid secretes by the adrenal glands.

Effect of Thyroid Hormone on Sexual Function. For normal sexual function, thyroid secretion needs to be approximately normal. In men, lack of thyroid hormone is likely to cause loss of libido; whereas great excesses of the hormone sometimes cause impotence. A hypothyroid woman, like a man, is likely to have greatly decreased libido.

In women, lack of thyroid hormone often causes menorrhagia and polymenorrhea, that is respectively, excessive and frequent menstrual bleeding. Yet, strangely enough, in other women thyroid lack may cause irregular periods and occasionally even amenorrhea.

To make the picture still more confusing, in the hyperthyroid woman, oligomenorrhea, which means "greatly reduced bleeding," is common, and occasionally amenorrhea results.

The action of thyroid hormone on the gonads cannot be pinpointed to a specific function but probably results from a combination of direct metabolic effects on the gonads, as well as excitatory and inhibitory feedback effects operating through the anterior pituitary hormones that control the sexual functions.

Appendix B
Mechanisms of Thyroid Hormone
Disruption by Synthetic Chemicals

There are many steps in the chemical reactions required to properly utilize thyroid hormones. The following chart is an overview of these different steps and the synthetic chemicals that disrupt them.

See Table 8 on the next page.

Table 8   **Synthetic Chemicals that Interfere with the Production,
                   Transport, and Metabolism of Thyroid Hormone.**

Thyroid mechanism and interfering chemical

Uptake of iodide by thyroid gland
2,4-D (137)
3-Amino-1,2,4-triazole (138,139)
Aldrin(140)
Amitrole (141, 142)
Aroclor (141, 142)
1,2-Dihydroxybenzene (catechol)(146)
4-Chlororesorcinol (146)
Clofentezine (141)
o-Cresol (146)
p-Cresol (146)
Cythion (96, 147)
1,3-Dihydroxynaphthalene (146)
1,5-Dihydroxynaphthalene (146)
2,3-Dihydroxynaphthalene (146)
2,7-Dihydroxynaphthalene (146)
2,4-Dihydroxybenzaldehyde (146)
2,4-Dihydroxybenzoic acid (146)
Ethiozin (141)
Ethylene thiourea (141, 148)
Fipronil (141)
Hexachlorobenzene(149,150)
Hexadrin (147)
4-Hexylresorcinol (146)
1,3,4-Trihydroxybenzene (hydroxyquinoI)
   (146)
Hydroxyquinol triacetate(146)
Lead (151)
Mancozeb (152)
Mercuric chloride (153,154)
3-Methylcholanthrene (143, 155)
Methylmercuric chloride (154)
Methylaparthion (156)
2-Methylresorcinol (146)
Mull-Soy (157)
Nabam (140)
5-Methylresorcinol (orcinol) (146)
Pendimethalin (141)
Pentachloronitrobenzene (141)
Phenobarbital (143)
Phenol (146)
1,3,5-Trihydroxybeozene (phloroglucinol)
   (146)
Polybrominated biphenyls (158)
Pregnenolone-16α-carbonitrile (143)
Propylthiouracil (139, 158)
1,2,3-Trihydroxybenzene pyrogallol) (146)
Pyrimenthanil (141)
1,3-Dihyroxybenzene(resorcinol) (146)
o-Hydroxybenzyl alcohol (saligenin) (146)
Selenium (151)
Thiocyanate (141)

Sodium/iodide symporter
Perchlorate (94, 159)
Perrhenate (159)

Serum protein-bound iodide level
2,4-D (137)
2,4-Dinitrophenol (96)
3-Methylcholanthrene (155)
Amitrole (142)
Aroclor 1254 (144)
Cython (95, 147)
Malathion (160)
Mancozeb (152)
Mercuric chloride (153)

o,p'-DDD (161,162)
Hexadrin (147)

Thyroid peroxidase action—general information
Amitrole (141)
Ammonia (154)
Ethylene thiouree (141)
Fipronil (141)
Mancozeb (141)
4,4'-Methylenedianiline (141)
Thiocyante (141)

Thyroid peroxidase action—oxidation of iodide
Aminotriazole (97, 164)
Ammonia (163)
Cadmium chloride (163, 165)
Endosulfan (166)
Ethylene thiourea (98)
1,2,3,4,5,6-Hexachlorocyclohexane (lindane) (167)
Malathion (167)
Mancozeb (152)
Mercury chloride (165)
Methamizole (97)
Polybrominated biphenyls (158)
Thiourea (166)

Thyroid peroxidase action—iodination of tyrosine
Polybrominated biphenyls (158)

Binding to thyroglobulin
o,p'-DDD (161)
Pentachlorophenol (168)

Binding to transthyretin
Bromoxynil (3.5-bibromo-4-hydroxybenzonitril)
   (99)
4-(Chloro-o-tolyloxy) acetic acid (99)
4-(4-Chloro-2-methylphenoxy) butyric acid (99)
Chlorophenol (99, 169)
Chloroxuron (99)
2,4-D (99)
2,4-Dicholorophenoxybutric acid (99)
Dioxtylpthalete (99)
o,p'-DDD (99)
p,p'-DDD(99)
2,3-Dichlorophenol (99, 169)
2,4-Dichlorophenol (99)
2,6-Dichlorophenol (99, 169, 170)
2-(2.4-Dicholorophenoxy) propionic acid
   [dichloroprop] (99)
1,1,1-Trichloro-2,2-bis(chlorophenol) ethanol
   [difocol] (99)
2,4-Dinitrophenol (99)
2,4-Dinitro-6-methyphenol (99)
Ethyl-bromophos (99)
Ethyl-parathion (99)
2-(2,4,5-Trichlorophenoxy) propionic acid
   [fenoprop] (99)
HexachIorobenzene (99)
Hexachlorophene (99, 169)
2-Hydroxybiphenyl (99)
4-Hydroxybiphenyl (99, 169)
Lindane (99)
Linuron (99)
Malathion (99)
Pentachlorophenol (99, 169, 170)
Phenol (169)

Pyrogallol (99)
2,4,5-Trichlorophenoxyacetic acid (99)
1,4-Tetrachlorophenol (99, 170)
PCB-77 (99, 105, 169)
Trichloroacetic acid (99)
2,3,4-Trichlorophenol (170)
2,4,5-Trichlorophenol (99, 169, 170)
2,4,6-Trichlorophenol (99, 170)
2,4,5-Trichlorophenoxyacetic acid
   methyl ester (99)

Binding to albumin
Pentachlorophenol (169)

**Catabolism of T4 or T3: type I or II
5'-deiodinase**
3,3',4,4',5,5'-Hexachlorobiphenyl (107)
3-Methylcholanthrene (171, 172)
Aminotriazole (106)
Amiodarone (94, 172)
Aroclor 1254 (109)
Cadmium chloride (173)
Diphrmylthiohydantoin (141,172)
Dimethoate (100, 174)
Fenvalerate (175,176)
Hexachlorobenzene (102)
Lead (177)
Phenobarbital (172)
Propylthiouracil (172)
PCB 77 (107, 171)
TCDD (171, 178)

Glucuronidation of T4/T3
Acetochlor (141)
Aroclor 1254 (109, 143-145, 179)
3,4-Benzpyrene (180)
Clofentenzine (141)
Clofibrate (141)
DDT (144)
Fenbuconazole (141)
3,3',4,4',5,5'-Hexabromobiphenyl (101)
Hexachlorobenzene (102, 183)
2,3,3',4,4',5-Hexachlorobiphenyl (182)
3,3',4,4',5,5'-Hexachlorobiphenyl (107)
3-Methylcholanthrene (141, 143, 155,
   171, 179)
Pendimethalin (141)
PCB 126 (108, 182)
Phenobarbital (141, 143, 172, 180,
   181, 183)
Polybrominated biphenyls (184)
PCBs (141)
Pregnenolone-16α-carbonitrile (141,
   143, 179)
Promadiamine (141)
Pyrimethanil (141)
PCB 77 (108, 171)
TCDD (108, 141, 178, 182)
Thiazopyr (141)

**Catabolism and biliary elimination of T4/
T3 in the liver**
Aroclor 1254 (144, 145)
3,4-Benzopyrene (180)
DDT (144)
Hexachlorobenzene (102)
3-Methylcholanthrene (155)
Phenobabital (180, 183)
Polybrominated biphenyls (184)

Abbreviations: 2,4-D 2,4-dichlorophenoxyacetic acid; DDD 1-1dichloro-2, 2-histo-chlorophenyllethane.

Source: Howdeshell K. A model of the development of the brain as a construct
of the thyroid system. *Environmental Health Perspectives*. 2002. 110(supp 3):337-8.

References

1   Heidenreich PA, Trogdon JG, Khavjou OA, Forecasting the future of cardiovascular disease in the united states: a policy statement from the American Heart Association. *Circulation*. 2011; 123:933-944.

   The World Health Bank Web site. Health Expenditure, Total (% of GDP). Available at: http://data.worldbank.org/indicator/SH.XPD.TOTL.ZS. Accessed November 18, 2013.

   Wikipedia Web site. List of countries by military expenditures. Available at: en.wikipedia.org/wiki/List_of_countries_by_military_expenditures. Accessed December 1, 2013.

2   Strong JP, McGill HC. The pediatric aspects of atherosclerosis. *Journal Atherosclerosis Research*. 1969; 9:251.

3   Barnes B. Etiology and treatment of lowered resistance to upper respiratory infection. *Federation Proceedings*. 1953; 12:10.

4   Barnes BO. *Heart Attack Rareness in Thyroid–Treated Patients*. Springfield, IL: Charles C. Thomas; 1972.

5   Barnes BO, Ratzenhofer M, Gisi R. The role of natural consequences in the changing death patterns. *Journal American of the American Geriatrics Society*. 1974; 22:176.

6   Heidenreich PA, Albert NM, Allen LA, et al. Forecasting the impact of heart failure in the United States: a policy statement from the American Heart Association. *Circ Heart Fail*. 2013. 6(3):606-619. doi: 10.1161/HHF.0b013e318291329a. Epub 2013 Apr 24.

7   Emory Healthcare Web site. Heart Failure Statistics. Available at: www.emoryhealthcare.org/heart-failure/learn-about-heart-failure/statistics.html. Accessed November 18, 2013.

8   Barnes BO. *Heart Attack Rareness in Thyroid–Treated Patients*. Springfield, IL: Charles C. Thomas; 1972.

   Barnes BO. *Solved: The Riddle of Heart Attacks*. Trumbull, CT: The Broda O. Barnes M.D. Research Foundation; 1976. Page 19.

   Barnes B, Galton L. *Hypothyroidism: The Unsuspected Illness*. New York: Harper and Row Publishers; 1976.

   Barnes BO, Barnes CW. *Hope for Hypoglycemia*. Revised Ed. America Book Company; 1999.

9 Fahr G. Myxedema heart. *JAMA*. 1925; 84(5):345-349.

10 American Diabetes Association Web site. Diabetes Statistics. Available at: www.diabetes.org/diabetes-basics/diabetes-statistics/. Accessed November 18, 2013.

11 Barnes BO. *Thyroid Therapy I, II, III* (Audio Tapes) Copies available through The Broda O. Barnes M.D. Research Foundation (www.brodabarnes.org or 203 261-2101).

12 Eaton CD. Co-existence of hypothyroidism with diabetes mellitus. *J Mich State Med Soc*. 1954; 53(10, Part 1):1101.

13 Kulacz R, Levy TE. *The Roots of Disease: Connecting Dentistry and Medicine*. Xlibris; 2002.
    Tennant J. *Healing is Voltage: The Handbook*. 3rd ed. CreateSpace Independent Publishing Platform; 2010. Available at: 972-580-1156.
    Meinig GE. *Root Canal Cover Up*. 9th ed. Price Pottenger Nutrition; 2008.
    Ewing D. *Let the Tooth Be Known . . . Are Your Teeth Making You Sick?* Holistic Health Alternatives; 1998.

14 Barnes B, Galton L. *Hypothyroidism: The Unsuspected Illness*. New York: Harper and Row Publishers; 1976.

15 NAH - National Academy of Hypothyroidism Web site. Deiodinases: Understanding Local Control of Thyroid Hormones (Deiodinases Function and Activity). Available at: http://nahypothyroidism.org/deiodinases/. Accessed January 2, 2013.

16 Tennant J. *Healing is Voltage: The Handbook*. 3rd ed. CreateSpace Independent Publishing Platform; 2010. Available at: 972-580-1156.

17 Hurxthal, I.M. Blood cholesterol and thyroid disease. *Archives Internal Medicine*. 1934; 53:762.

18 Barnes BO. *Solved: The Riddle of Heart Attacks*. Trumbull, CT: The Broda O. Barnes M.D. Research Foundation; 1976. Page 19.

19 Cheron RG, Kaplan MM, Larsen PR. Physiological and pharmacological influences on thyroxine to 3,5,3'-triiodothyronine conversion and nuclear 3,5,3'-triiodthyroidne binding in rat anterior pituitary. *J Clin Invest*. 1979; 64:1402-1414.

20 Tennant J. *Healing is Voltage: The Handbook*. 3rd ed. CreateSpace Independent Publishing Platform; 2010. Available at: 972-580-1156.
    Starr M. *Hypothyroidism Type 2: The Epidemic*. New Voice Publications, Irvine, CA. 2005, revised 2013.

21 Starr M. *Hypothyroidism Type 2: The Epidemic*. New Voice Publications, Irvine, CA. 2005, revised 2013. Basal Temperature pages 12-13.

22 Barnes BO. Basal temperature versus basal metabolism. *JAMA*. 1942; 119:1072-1073.

23 Starr M. *Hypothyroidism Type 2: The Epidemic*. New Voice Publications, Irvine, CA. 2005, revised 2013.

24 Sonkin L. Therapeutic trials with thyroid hormones in chemically normal thyroid patients with myofascial pain and complaints suggesting mild thyroid insufficiency. *Journal of Back and Musculoskeletal Rehabilitation*. 1997; 8(83):85.

25 U.S. National Library of Medicine Web site. A.D.A.M. Medical Encyclopedia. Chronic thyroiditis (Hashimoto's disease). Available at: www.ncbi.nlm.nih.gov/pubmedhealth/PMH0001409/. Accessed November 18, 2013.

26 Environmental Working Group Web site. Video: 10 Americans. Available at: www.ewg.org/news/videos/10-americans. Accessed November 18, 2013.

27 Lisser H, Escamilla RF. *Atlas of Clinical Endocrinology: Including Text of Diagnosis and Treatment*. St. Louis: C.V. Mosby Company. 1957.

28 Kirsch I, Deacon BJ, Huedo-Medina TB, Scoboria A, Moore TJ, Johnson BT. Initial severity and antidepressant benefits: a meta-analysis of data submitted to the Food and Drug Administration. *PLoS Med*. 2008; 5(2):e45. doi: 10.1371/journal.pmed.0050045.

29 Roberts HJ. *Aspartame Disease: An Ignored Epidemic*. Sunshine Sentinel Pr, Inc. 2001.
    The Huffington Post Web site. Gennet R. Donald Rumsfeld and the Strange History of Aspartame. Available at: www.huffingtonpost.com/robbie-gennet/donald-rumsfeld-and-the-s_b_805581.html. Accessed December 8, 2013.
    Wikipedia Web site. Donald Rumsfeld. Available at: http://en.wikipedia.org/wiki/Donald_Rumsfeld. Accessed December 8, 2013.

Index